A Guide to Establishing Programs for Assessing Outcomes in Clinical Settings

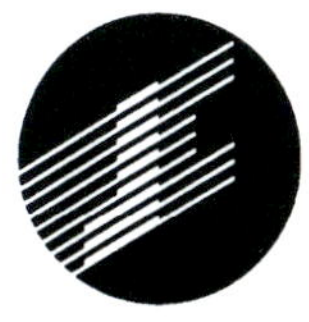

JOINT COMMISSION

CONTRIBUTORS

Allyson Ross Davies, PhD, is senior program advisor, Measurement and Monitoring Initiative, New England Medical Center, Boston.

M. Anne Thomas Doyle, MA, is a principal in Doyle Consulting, Minneapolis. Formerly she was the vice president of strategic development, Park Nicollet Medical Foundation, Minneapolis.

David Lansky, PhD, is the regional director for clinical information for Sisters of Providence Health System, Oregon, and directs its Center for Outcomes Research and Education.

Wilmer Rutt, MD, is the founder of the Center for Clinical Effectiveness, Henry Ford Health System, Detroit.

Marcia O. Stevic, PhD, RN, is a health care research consultant. Formerly she was the director of quality research for the Cleveland Clinic Foundation, Cleveland.

John B. Doyle, PhD, is a principal in Doyle Consulting, Minneapolis.

Joint Commission Mission

The mission of the Joint Commission on Accreditation of Healthcare
Organizations is to improve the quality of health care provided to
the public.

The work described in this book was supported by a grant from the
New England Medical Center Incorporated through the auspices of the
Henry J. Kaiser Family Foundation.

Discussion of legal issues in this work is not intended to be, and should
not be construed to be, a substitute for legal advice. Legal advice can only
be obtained from a licensed attorney who knows applicable law in the
relevant jurisdiction.

Printed in the U.S.A.   1 2 3 4 5

Requests for permission to reprint or make copies of any part
of this book should be mailed to:
Permissions Editor
Department of Publications
Joint Commission on Accreditation of Healthcare Organizations

ISBN: 0-86688-377-0
Library of Congress Catalog Card Number: 93-80586

Contents

Foreword

Today's health care environment is characterized by ever-increasing and powerful pressures to contain costs and improve quality. This environment mandates the measurement of patient health care outcomes and the processes used to achieve them. The goal of all health care services is to achieve good patient outcomes as measured by such factors as physiological status, functional status, and freedom from physical and psychological pain. The information derived from measuring patient care outcomes and processes, including information about patient satisfaction as well as the costs associated with the outcomes of care, is important to all involved. Such information is key to health care organizations and professionals as they strive to improve performance. It is valuable to patients and their clinicians as they make decisions about care strategies and delivery, and it is of use to purchasers who in today's environment must identify efficient providers of quality health care services.

The Joint Commission's aim is now, and always has been, to encourage and help health care organizations measure and improve their performance through the use of our standards, accreditation process, educational programs, consultation services, and publications. Because of our commitment to the measurement of outcomes and processes of care, we are particularly pleased to present *A Guide to Establishing Programs for Assessing Outcomes in Clinical Settings* to the health care field. This publication relates the experiences of, and offers suggestions from, leaders in the implementation of outcomes assessment programs at five health care organizations: Cleveland Clinic Foundation, Cleveland; Henry Ford Health System, Detroit; New England Medical Center Hospitals, Boston; Park Nicollet Medical Foundation, Minneapolis; and Sisters of Providence Health System, Oregon, Portland.

Under a grant from the Functional Outcomes Program of the New England Medical Center, the directors of the health outcomes assessment programs for these five organizations met to discuss their experiences and reach consensus on principles that would be useful to other health care organizations striving to develop outcomes assessment programs. Their observations and advice are confirmed by the experiences of hospitals that have participated with the Joint Commission in developing and testing our Indicator Measurement System. The IMSystem is a component of the Joint Commission Agenda for Change, a major initiative designed to provide health care organizations with comparative information about their outcomes and processes. This information should prove critical to improving organizational performance.

The experience and advice of this publication's authors will help health care organizations in implementing outcomes assessment programs and participating in reference databases such as the Joint Commission's IMSystem.

Paul M. Schyve, MD
Senior Vice President
Joint Commission on Accreditation of Healthcare Organizations

Preface

There is an idea, shared by many providers and consumers of health care, that patient outcomes should be evaluated as part of routine care. This book represents the early experiences of a handful of health care organizations trying to transform the idea into practice.

In May 1992, under a grant from the Functional Outcomes Program of the New England Medical Center, we, the directors of five major health outcomes assessment programs, formed the Outcomes Implementation Network and began meeting to discuss shared experiences in implementation. By comparing and documenting our experiences as early adopters, we hope this book can help other health care organizations wishing to implement an effective outcomes effort.

We agreed to focus our discussions on seven critical issues in implementing an outcomes assessment program:

- Organization;
- Project management;
- Financing;
- Education, training, and awareness raising;
- Ethical and legal concerns;
- Interinstitutional issues; and
- Demonstrating value.

Each participating program director prepared an extended outline and led discussions on one or more of these seven topics.

An independent editor documented the proceedings of meetings and integrated them into position papers. These expanded position papers, augmented and modified by the network members, are presented here as book chapters in the hope that they will help others organize and implement programs for measuring, monitoring, and managing the outcomes of care.

This book will be of interest primarily to those who are launching or managing an outcomes assessment initiative within a health care organization. This is not a how-to manual for putting together an outcomes project. The focus is more exploratory than prescriptive. It is also not an academic treatise; the writing style reflects the informal nature of our conversations. Taken together, these chapters provide a summary of the major issues that a health care setting is likely to confront as it seeks to implement an outcomes initiative.

Throughout our discussions we sought to establish a consensus among network members regarding recommended best practices for implementing an outcomes assessment effort. In reaching consensus we tried our best to anticipate how our experiences might translate to organizations of varying types and sizes. These consensus positions are interspersed throughout the text.

The network meetings were the first opportunity for us to discuss important issues with colleagues in a structured format. It became clear that, in this evolving realm of outcomes assessment, consensus is neither clear-cut nor static. Where disagreement persists we have tried to present the major alternatives. As methods improve and as we gain more experience, many of our opinions from late 1992 are likely to change over time. The intent is to stimulate further thought and interaction rather than to proclaim the "right" way to do things. We enthusiastically encourage others to experiment with alternative approaches and to share their experiences with us.

One main objective was to develop a brief and practical

"Organizational Implementation Workbook" that highlights many of the key decisions and actions that need to be addressed in implementing an outcomes assessment initiative. We encourage readers to refer to the workbook (see page 139) as they develop their strategies and work plans.

We would like to express our appreciation to Dr Ed Schor and Dr Al Tarlov of the Functional Outcomes Program at New England Medical Center for supporting this project. Thanks also to Dr Rick Ward of Henry Ford Health System and Julie Sanderson Austin of American Group Practice Association for their helpful comments on earlier drafts, and to Jayne Hoese of Park Nicollet Medical Foundation for her excellent technical support in preparing the manuscript.

We hope this book helps advance the outcomes movement as it makes the difficult but rewarding advancement from promise to reality.

Allyson Ross Davies, PhD, New England Medical Center, Boston

M. Anne Thomas Doyle, MA, Park Nicollet Medical Foundation,
Minneapolis

David Lansky, PhD, Sisters of Providence Health System, Oregon,
Portland

Wilmer Rutt, MD, Henry Ford Health System, Detroit

Marcia O. Stevic, PhD, RN, Cleveland Clinic Foundation, Cleveland

John B. Doyle, PhD, Minneapolis (Editor)

Executive Summary

The health care system faces major demands for change from policymakers, purchasers, insurers, administrators, clinicians, and patients. In looking for solutions, attention is shifting to the importance of understanding the outcomes of care.

Health outcomes go beyond traditional measures of mortality and complications to include the patient's physiology, signs and symptoms, functional status, and well-being. An outcomes assessment effort focuses on measuring these constructs, monitoring patients over time, and giving clinicians feedback about results to help them optimize the process of care.

The primary mission of an outcomes assessment initiative is to help bring about a shift toward an empirical basis for routine clinical decision making. In a sense, outcomes assessment is analogous to industrial research and development: research in support of operations. However, it also represents a new way of thinking about health care. Leadership, communication, and education are as important as technical proficiency in implementing an outcomes assessment program in a health care setting.

Outcomes assessment should be part of a comprehensive strategy. Those who plan and implement a program should keep the larger vision in mind as they launch specific outcomes projects. They should also plan for the transition of the outcomes initiative from small-scale demonstration projects to integration throughout the care system.

ORGANIZATION

In launching an outcomes assessment effort, it is best to identify
and build on existing capabilities and related activities within the
organization. To get underway, an outcomes initiative needs a few
committed clinicians, sufficient financial and technical resources
to conduct a pilot project, at least a moderate level of support and
interest from top management, and a catalyst with vision and
influence to lead the charge and coalesce the other ingredients
into an initial project.

Organizational motivation for launching an outcomes initiative is typically based on a combination of factors: purchaser
demand, continuous quality improvement, and scientific interest.
To achieve its potential, the outcomes program should set realistic
short-term objectives within the context of the organization's
overall goals. Strategic planning should recognize the importance
of bottom-up support in bringing about widespread change.

An outcomes assessment program should provide both
technical expertise and leadership. Its initial placement within the
organizational structure is likely to be determined more by
opportunity than by logic. Over time, the technical expertise is
likely to become centralized and possibly merged with other
similar activities. Responsibility for most of the ongoing implementation will shift to the clinicians. Throughout the stages of
organizational evolution, the importance of leadership for the
larger mission must remain paramount.

Leadership and overall direction are the key responsibilities of
the outcomes program manager. Staffing, either in-house or
through consultants, should cover the core functions of an
outcomes assessment project, discussed more fully in Chapter 2,
Project Management.

PROJECT MANAGEMENT

Most of the work in implementing outcomes assessment is concentrated in managing individual projects. Begin with projects that are less difficult: limited in scope and objectives, with minimal technical or logistical challenges, and administered within a single clinical department. A project coordinator should serve as task manager and liaison between medical administration, clinicians and their staff, and the outcomes assessment technical personnel.

There should be agreement among all key participants regarding the central purpose of the project. Instruments for measuring outcomes and related constructs should be brief and easy to administer; start with existing measurement tools wherever possible. The project protocol should be designed to minimize not only the logistical burden on clinicians but also the disruption to patient care flow and patients themselves.

A significant proportion of the overall effort goes into achieving efficient data collection. Protocols should specify when data are to be collected (during an encounter, at specified intervals), from whom to collect it (patients, clinicians), and how to collect it (in person, by mail, by chart review). Similarly, tactics for data entry into a database vary according to when, by whom, and how the data should be entered. A data quality control method should be established. Generally speaking, it is best if the clinicians and their staff eventually assume ownership of these aspects of data management.

An outcomes database, whether a stand-alone program or part of a centralized information system, should play a supporting role in outcomes assessment. Build or buy the database that best supports the organization's data management plan; do not build the plan *around* the database. Linkages to other data sets (for example, cost, utilization, satisfaction) can help maximize the value and efficiency of the outcomes initiative.

Statistical data analyses should be focused on addressing the purposes of the project. Analyses must be presented in ways that all project participants can understand. Success is achieved if clinicians and/or administrators actually use the findings to evaluate and improve the effectiveness of the care process.

FINANCING

The costs of organizing and administering an outcomes assessment effort can be allocated to three broad categories: start-up, technology development, and ongoing operations. Generally speaking, the greater the up-front investment in planning and infrastructure, the lower the operating costs later on. Budgeting for each cost category depends on the anticipated scale of implementation, the technological state of the art, and potential synergies to be achieved by integrating outcomes assessment with related activities.

Various sources of external funding may be available for outcomes work. However, if outcomes assessment is to become regarded as part of the care delivery process, an organizational commitment to internal funding must eventually be made. Program managers should plan the transition from designated funding for specific outcomes projects to self-funding from clinical operations.

EDUCATION, TRAINING, AND AWARENESS RAISING

The outcomes technical staff should acquire a shared understanding of outcomes assessment and a commitment to the mission. Each staff member should become familiar with the various technical skills required to carry out an outcomes project. Outcomes staff and project support staff need specific skills training for routine activities such as data entry and responding to inquiries about the program.

For clinicians to incorporate an outcomes perspective into their practice, they need a general orientation to quantitative thinking. Outcomes projects provide a "living laboratory" for acquiring key concepts experientially. Those who are already enthusiastic about outcomes can benefit from content-rich exposure to new ideas and methods. Research-oriented clinicians are willing to consider outcomes assessment if it generates data relevant to issues they are already pursuing. The rest, including skeptics and those too busy to participate in outcomes projects, need more information about the increasing importance and relevance of outcomes assessment. There should be a structured forum in which the strategic aspects of the outcomes assessment program are made known to all the clinicians.

Administrators need continual awareness raising about the importance of outcomes information and the activities underway within and outside the organization. New methods are being investigated for giving patients feedback about their outcomes. The health care organization should take a role in teaching insurers and purchasers to be responsible consumers of outcomes information.

ETHICAL AND LEGAL CONCERNS

Patients, clinicians, and administrators have confidentiality concerns with respect to outcomes data. Health care organizations should establish consensual criteria for deciding who can have access to which outcomes data and reports, and in what form the information will be made available. Data access policies should be informed by legal opinion.

Patients should be informed of how and when the outcomes information they provide will be used in the care process. Patients should assume responsibility for responding to outcomes questionnaires with as much diligence as any other questions they may be asked during the course of treatment.

Outcomes data are subject to various sources of distortion, including lapses in data quality control, methodological biases, and *gaming the system* (see page 115 for an explanation of systems gaming). Outcomes program managers should prevent and correct such controllable sources of error.

INTERINSTITUTIONAL ISSUES

Health care organizations often need access to methodological resources that are unavailable internally. Research literature is a good starting point for selecting or modifying measurement instruments. Also, software vendors have begun entering the market with outcomes database management systems. However, there should be a national center or clearinghouse to provide technical support to outcomes assessment projects.

Opportunities exist for sharing practical experience in outcomes implementation. A number of conferences, seminars, and newsletters on outcomes have appeared on the scene. Outcomes interest groups are needed as a semiformal mechanism for promoting interinstitutional learning.

The pooling of outcomes data from multiple sites offers an opportunity to accumulate large data sets for detailed analyses and to compare results of care across institutions. The benefits of pooling must be weighed against the added logistical complexities involved. Many of the advantages of data pooling can be attained by sites agreeing to compare results of internal projects with one another.

DEMONSTRATING VALUE

Outcomes assessment is of value to patients, policymakers, purchasers, administrators, and clinicians. Nevertheless, there are three significant obstacles to demonstrating value: the cost of development and implementation, fear by clinicians of inappropriate use of the data, and indifference.

Outcomes projects must begin to document their impact on patient opinion, clinician perceptions, and the impact on care processes. Significant effort must be devoted to communicating, especially to clinicians, the value of outcomes initiatives. To maximize impact and minimize costs, outcomes assessment should work collaboratively with other internal efforts to improve the quality and efficiency of care.

Introduction

The health care system is facing a number of major challenges.

- Policymakers want efficient and effective allocation of resources to improve the health of the population.
- Purchasers are demanding accountability and value for their dollar.
- Insurers and HMOs, dissatisfied with the micromanagerial aspects of traditional managed care, are looking for a more effective, collaborative, and economical basis for working with providers.
- Administrators are struggling to import industrial quality management ideas and methods into the clinic and the hospital.
- Clinicians, tired of the second-guessing, post-hoc inspection, and seemingly arbitrary practice parameters imposed by insurers and regulators, want to establish a scientific basis for determining what "best practices" really are.
- Innovative administrators and clinicians want to develop an automated medical record that affords a more systematic method for collecting, storing, and analyzing patient data.
- Patients want to communicate effectively with their physicians, make informed choices about their own care, and be assured of the best possible care.

In responding to these challenges, an increasing number of health care professionals and institutions have begun to look systematically at patient outcomes.

WHAT ARE OUTCOMES?

An outcome is the result of a process. A good outcome is a result that achieves the goal of the process. There are a number of goals of the health care process, many of which directly relate to patients' health.

- Avoiding adverse effects of care (for example, premature death, secondary infections, return hospitalizations). This sort of defensive goal has been a focus of attention for traditional quality assurance programs.
- Improving the patient's physiological status (for example, blood pressure, blood gas readings, degree of arterial blockage). These hard indicators are usually more important to the physician than to the patient.
- Reducing the patient's signs and symptoms (for example, shortness of breath, pain). These are indicators that the patient can observe and that probably bring the patient to the physician in the first place.
- Improving the patient's functional status and well-being (for example, ability to climb stairs, anxiety about one's health, ability to work). These indicators, directly observable by the patient, reflect the impact of health on the activities of daily living.

There are other goals of health care that are not directly health related:

- Achieving patient satisfaction (for example, with the facilities, the attitude of the staff);
- Minimizing the cost of care (for example, by avoiding unnecessary diagnosis and treatment); and

■ Maximizing revenues (for example, by recruiting new patients).

Although these goals are important, the focus of this book is on health-related outcomes, particularly symptom reduction and health status improvement. This emphasis on health outcomes represents the shared belief among the Outcomes Implementation Network that health care should be patient centered, and that the patient is the best judge of outcome.

WHY OUTCOMES?

A number of paths continue to lead to this increasing attention to outcomes.

1. **Public policy** has targeted health care as the number one priority for reform in the United States. The spiraling costs of care have not led to a measurable improvement in the overall health and well-being of the population. The public outcry for cost containment must be balanced against the equally strong demand for universal access to care. The measurement of outcomes on a national scale can help establish standards of effectiveness for a minimum package of universal health benefits.

2. **Purchaser demand** has become more sophisticated. In addition to cost containment, purchasers are looking for demonstrable value of the health care dollars they spend. Several employer coalitions and state governments have begun to require providers to collect outcomes data. In some instances they have committed themselves to buying selectively, based on the ability of providers to measure and improve outcomes.

3. **Quality assurance** in health care has traditionally focused on identifying the exceptionally poor outcomes: mortality and morbidity. Explanations are sought after the fact

through an investigatory process, typically involving chart reviews and interrogation of individual clinicians. It gradually became clear that this sort of problem-centered approach fails to identify opportunities for process improvement. Continuous monitoring of outcomes is needed to obtain the data needed for system change.

The introduction of continuous quality improvement (CQI) into health care promises to integrate outcomes assessment more closely into the care delivery process. In particular, CQI emphasizes the

- ever-repeating cycle of improvement: plan a process, carry it out, study the outcome, identify opportunities for process improvement, and act on the results;
- need for clinicians themselves to assume responsibility for quality control and improvement; and
- importance of meeting and exceeding patient expectations with respect to satisfaction and improved health status.

4. **Clinical research** has historically relied on the randomized controlled trial. This methodology can demonstrate the *efficacy* of treatment under ideal circumstances; it cannot demonstrate *effectiveness* in routinely delivered care. Multisite observational studies have shown large variations in outcome between and within sites. Researchers, administrators, and clinicians are increasingly recognizing the importance of observational outcome studies.

Another trend in outcomes research is the increasing attention to health status. The success of treatment has usually been measured in terms of "hard" physiological indicators and lab tests. Now the focus has broadened to include the patient's perspective on quality of care, as indicated by improved well-being and functional status.

5. **The computerized medical record** promises improved efficiency in the collection, storage, retrieval, and use of clinical information. To achieve its full potential, the medical record should be able to function as a database for clinical research and quality assessment activities. Consequently, clinicians are attempting to record patient information, including patient outcomes, in a more systematic fashion.

Our efforts to establish outcomes assessment activities are shaped by these trends.

consensus

Among the most important reasons for establishing an outcomes assessment initiative in a health care setting are

- to describe, in quantitative terms, the impact of routinely delivered care on patients' lives;
- to establish a more accurate and reliable basis for clinical decision making by clinicians and patients; and
- to evaluate the effectiveness of care and identify opportunities for improvement.

Enhancing patients' quality of life is the primary incentive; marketing or administrative motivations should be secondary.

MEASUREMENT, MONITORING, AND MANAGEMENT

Our work in outcomes assessment (see note on next page) can be summarized in terms of three core activities:

- **Outcomes measurement** (the *systematic, quantitative observation, at a point in time,* of outcome indicators);

- **Outcomes monitoring** (the *repeated measurement over time* of outcome indicators in a manner that permits causal inferences about what [patient characteristics, care processes, resources] produced the observed patient outcomes); and

- **Outcomes management** (the *use of information and knowledge* gained from outcome monitoring to achieve optimal patient outcomes through improved clinical decision making and service delivery).

At this stage the measurement and monitoring functions take up most of our time and effort. Managing outcomes is accomplished by managing the care process that generates the outcomes: primarily the domain of the clinicians and the organizations in which they work. With regard to outcomes management, the job of an outcomes team is *feedback*—to provide clinicians with useful, meaningful, and accurate data and help them interpret the data as they analyze and modify the care process.

NOTE: Throughout this book the term *outcomes assessment* refers collectively to outcomes measurement, monitoring, and feedback.

META-ISSUES

The network was charged with documenting its shared experiences in implementing outcomes assessment in the real world. Most of our observations are organized by topic in the chapters that follow. Some issues, however, transcended topical boundaries, influencing discussion and consensus at various points. These *meta-issues*, outlined briefly here, help define a broader context for the implementation of outcomes assessment.

Research or Operations?

How does outcomes assessment fit into the health care system? There is a traditional split in health care between research and operations.

Research, roughly defined, is an activity directed toward discovering and disseminating new knowledge. Methods have been standardized for design, measurement, data collection, and data analysis. Research projects are limited in scope and duration, and directed toward testing hypotheses. To ensure unambiguous results, clinical research projects are usually administered under controlled conditions, with precisely defined criteria for patient inclusion and carefully specified treatment protocols.

Operations are the core activities involved in running a business. Operations are ongoing functions, directed by distinct organizational units, funded from business revenues. The delivery of care is the main operations-level work of a group practice or hospital. Administrative functions, such as information systems and accounting, exist to support operations.

Outcomes assessment usually begins as a small-scale pilot project. As it proves itself and becomes visible in an organization, it must define its niche: Is it research or operations? Both the research and the operations paradigms capture some of the features of outcomes assessment while missing others. Research captures the analytical and developmental orientation of outcomes assessment and provides a methodological foundation for the work. However, the clinical researcher's historical preference for discrete studies under controlled conditions is not compatible with the continuous monitoring of outcomes in routine care. Likewise, we regard the insistence on hypothesis testing as too formal. Our analyses of outcomes data have been largely exploratory, descriptive, and predictive.

In its emphasis on continuous monitoring of routinely delivered care, outcomes assessment looks like an operations-level activity. We do want outcomes assessment to become a part of the ongoing work of health care organizations. However, *operations* connotes the sense that outcomes assessment is an administrative tool for managing the clinicians. We believe that an outcomes orientation is something not to be imposed on the clinicians, but to be initiated and "owned" by them.

consensus

> The mission of outcomes assessment is to help bring about a shift toward an empirical basis for routine clinical decision making. Outcomes assessment is closer to what in the industry is called *R&D,* which is research in support of operations. The intent is *to work with* clinicians in designing and implementing a new orientation to the work of health care.

The outcomes assessment effort cannot fulfill its mission by being isolated from clinical operations. It must seek input from the clinicians in accomplishing its measurement and monitoring functions. It must help clinicians use the data in improving clinical care to deliver the best possible patient outcomes.

A New Idea

Implementing an outcomes project requires technical expertise: in design, measurement, data management, and statistical analysis. But the outcomes assessment movement is more than a technology; it wants to present a new idea—that the routine collection and use of quantitative information in clinical decision making can improve the health care system. Disseminating the new idea and empowering clinicians to make the idea a reality are critical for an outcomes assessment initiative. Technical proficiency and logistical efficiency are important in implementation. At the same time, the larger vision must be communicated clearly and enthusiastically.

consensus

Tactics of implementation should exemplify the new idea. Clinicians should take ownership of outcomes projects from the beginning. As possible, technical experts should equip clinicians and their support staffs with the implementation skills needed to assume increasing responsibility for performing the work. Clinicians should be taught how to interpret results and how to use them in clinical practice. This empowerment strategy may reduce efficiency in implementation in the short run. Nevertheless, this strategy is essential if the larger mission of culture change is to succeed.

Strategy Versus Projects

Outcomes assessment is a component in a more comprehensive strategy for changing the delivery of health care. It can help establish an empirical basis for clinical decision making, patterns of care, and quality improvement. We find, however, that an outcomes strategy happens one project at a time. Should the strategic agenda dictate, top down, the nature and course of the projects? Or should the projects be paramount, so as to promote buy-in of participants throughout the health care organization? This tension between management and empowerment influences a number of implementation decisions.

consensus

"Think globally, act locally." Given the limited (but growing) state of the art in outcomes technology, fulfillment of the larger vision must occur incrementally through a series of projects. Implementers should keep the strategic direction in mind, but focus primarily on making each project run smoothly, rigorously, and with maximum buy-in from clinicians. Insights gained from each project can help refine the strategy from the bottom up.

Communication

An outcomes assessment effort lives in a climate of interdependence.

- It overlaps significantly in mission with clinical research and CQI.
- In planning and implementation, it requires close interaction with the clinicians.
- Its data-intensive nature gives it an important interface with information systems.
- Its role as a change agent means frequent interactions with the influence leaders of the health care community.

An outcomes assessment program needs to manage the organizational boundaries in fulfilling its mission. The key is communication.

consensus

As a new kid on the block in health care, outcomes assessment needs to be proactive in building an effective communication network. It is particularly important to manage the "white spaces" in the organizational chart; that is, to develop cross-organizational linkages. To induce culture change, informal communication channels are more important than formal structures.

Phasing

What is true of early implementation may not be true later. Some aspects of the work become more important over time, and others less so. The overall outcomes program evolves; each individual project undergoes its own maturation process.

Generally speaking, outcomes assessment implementation goes through predictable phases from:

- Smaller scale to larger scale;
- Developmental to operational;
- Demonstration to integration;
- Centralized to decentralized; and
- Measurement to monitoring to management.

Where appropriate, we have tried to identify phase-specific recommendations for implementation.

consensus

Directors of outcomes assessment initiatives should anticipate the phase transitions when planning programmatic activities.

Technology

In laying down the ground rules for the Outcomes Implementation Network, we agreed to focus our discussions and recommendations on organizational and implementation issues. Again and again, however, attention shifted to the technology of outcomes assessment—measurement instruments, data collection aids, database hardware and software, statistical analysis techniques, and reporting and feedback mechanisms. Not surprisingly, the emerging technology of outcomes assessment is inconsistent in quality and in breadth of applicability. Although improvements are occurring every day, technological limitations make implementation more difficult.

consensus

There should be a clearinghouse of information on technical concerns, to which health care organizations can contribute their experiences and from which they can obtain useful information. The idea of a clearinghouse is explored further in Chapter 6, Interinstitutional Issues.

1
Organization

Organizing an outcomes assessment effort in a clinic or hospital requires a combination of vision, commitment, technical skill, and hard work. Each of the organizations has pursued a different pathway in building its outcome program.

HISTORY: THE OUTCOMES IMPLEMENTATION NETWORK PROGRAMS

New England Medical Center (NEMC), Department of Quality Assessment (DQA), Boston

DQA was established in July 1988 and charged with creating and maintaining systems for monitoring (1) patient assessments of their functional status and well-being and (2) patients', family members', clinicians', and staffs' evaluations of the quality of care and services. DQA's mission captured the vision of NEMC's president and chief executive officer (CEO), who wanted to find out if such assessments, used primarily in health policy research and clinical trials, were "ready for prime time," that is, for including the patient's viewpoint among the information used to monitor and improve the quality of care provided by the hospital, from patient level to hospitalwide performance.

Work on developing a health outcomes assessment program

began in earnest in January 1990, supported by a three-year grant from the Functional Outcomes Program (then based at the Henry J. Kaiser Family Foundation). The primary purpose of the pilot program was to implement and test all features of a health outcomes measurement and monitoring system within an operating health care delivery organization; it stopped short of committing to the development of a hospitalwide system.

Early health outcomes assessment projects grew in response to interest expressed by clinicians in adding patient-based health status measures to their clinical practice and clinical research. By late 1992 the program included outcomes projects in end-stage renal disease, orthopedics (knee, spine), pain management, cardiology and cardiothoracic surgery, pediatric rheumatology, adult outpatient general medicine, and nursing functional status assessment. DQA's project support emphasizes development or adaptation of patient-based health assessment methods and feedback formats, and integration of data collection procedures into routine clinical workflow.

By mid-1992 the health outcomes assessment program had become an explicit part of NEMC's major organizational directives, and NEMC was engaged in developing strategic plans to build a hospitalwide system to support assessment efforts. In late 1992 NEMC announced the beginning of a major reorganization of care and services delivery into *care programs:* multidisciplinary, interdepartmental service delivery programs organized around the needs and conditions of similar groups of patients. At the same time, NEMC embarked on a Measurement and Monitoring Initiative (MMI) designed to provide the capability to measure and to monitor performance against standards for clinical outcomes, functional status and well-being, patient/customer satisfaction, and financial performance. The first coordinated outcomes monitoring system is being built to support the cardiac care program.

DQA's initial staff included a part-time director and a full-time all-purpose staff member with a combined clinical and health services research background. As of December 1992 staff consisted of the director of the health assessment team (also acting codirector of DQA), a project coordinator, three project assistants, a full-time programmer analyst and database administrator, a half-time systems coordinator, a half-time operations manager, and a half-time secretary. In December DQA's original director became cochair (with NEMC's chief financial officer) of the MMI effort. DQA, which originally reported jointly to NEMC's president and chief executive officer (on programmatic issues) and the chief operating officer (on operational and financial issues), now reports to the cochairs of the MMI program.

Park Nicollet Medical Foundation (PNMF), Outcomes Assessment Design and Development (OADD) Group, Minneapolis

The OADD Group was started in early 1989 within PNMF, a non-profit organization dedicated to research, education, and development for the improvement of health care. Although technically an independent organization, PNMF is closely associated with Park Nicollet Medical Center (PNMC), a large multispecialty group practice.

The OADD Group evolved from an outcomes-based initiative of the foundation's Arthritis Center. The Arthritis Center's outcomes assessment strategy included measures of health status and clinical indicators as part of routine care for patients with rheumatic diseases.

As local interest in outcomes assessment grew, top administration of PNMC requested that the Arthritis Center develop and manage a project exploring more broadly the feasibility and usefulness of outcomes assessment. Funded jointly for three years by PNMC and Blue Cross/Blue Shield of Minnesota, the "Outcomes Demonstration and Feasibility Project" focused primarily on three areas: total hip replacement in orthopedics, cataract surgery in ophthalmology, and all patients seen in rheumatology. Each project had a physician "champion" within the relevant department and was supported by PNMF outcomes staff.

At the beginning of 1993 PNMF's outcomes program was renamed the Outcomes Assessment Design and Development Group. Along with its historic emphasis on project implementation, the OADD Group has expanded its scope to include the design and development of methods for outcomes assessment. Seven outcomes projects have been launched, and work is now expanding beyond PNMC to include clinicians from other organizations.

The original 1989 outcomes assessment group was staffed part time by the executive director and administrative assistant of the Arthritis Center. By early 1993 staff resources included an implementation director, a technology director, a project manager, a project analyst, an instrumentation specialist, a project coordinator, data entry staff, and administrative support staff.

Sisters of Providence Health System, Oregon, Center for Outcomes Research and Education (CORE), Portland, Oregon

CORE was formed in 1989 at St. Vincent Hospital of Portland. Evolving within a long-standing cardiac surgery research group, CORE brought new emphases on patient health status and on the broader disease process. It then extended these methods to other clinical areas. By 1992 the program included outcomes projects in cardiological interventions, low back pain, neck and back surgery, total hip replacement, knee replacement, cataract surgery, and cholecystectomy.

Until 1992, each major CORE initiative was driven by the scientific and economic interests of one or two lead physicians, typically seeking data for quality improvement or for marketing their practice. St Vincent's parent health system, the Sisters of Providence Health System, Oregon, has given increasing weight to outcomes assessment as part of its strategic direction. In 1992 CORE was asked to assume operations of tumor registries in three hospitals and to convert them to "cancer information systems." CORE was also given responsibility for all patient satisfaction surveys and an annual survey of employee health status. In 1993 CORE moved from St Vincent Hospital to the parent system, with responsibilities for measuring quality and outcomes at all hospital facilities and within the new primary care division.

The initial CORE staff consisted of a biostatistician, two data management specialists, and a technical writer. As functional responsibility has grown, so has the staff. As of January 1993 the staff consisted of 4 PhD researchers, 6 research analysts, 11 data registrars, a systems manager, an operations manager, and a secretary. The center reports to a senior administrator with specific responsibilities within the multihospital system who also serves as CEO of one of the member hospitals.

Henry Ford Health System (HFHS), Center for Clinical Effectiveness (CCE), Detroit

In 1989 HFHS's medical leader asked a strategic question: "Where should we be going in outcomes management systems?" Several clinician leaders attended early developmental conferences sponsored by Dr Paul Ellwood and the InterStudy group. A two-hour seminar describing the basic concepts of outcomes management was offered to all clinical department chairpersons and/or representatives from their departments.

The first outcomes assessment project in diabetes mellitus was begun in 1990 under the leadership of two senior physicians. HFHS then joined a consortium of six group practices sponsored by the American Group Practice Association (AGPA) and

InterStudy. This group chose to study total hip replacement in each institution and to collect, analyze, and share data in a reasonably standardized way. Collection of data began on all patients receiving total hip replacements for one year starting April 1991. Subsequently AGPA has expanded the number of groups and the number of subjects so that now HFHS is participating in projects on total hip replacement, diabetes, cataract, and asthma. Additional projects under development include low back pain, management of prostatic hypertrophy, early diagnosis of prostatic cancer, and smoking cessation.

Clinical departments provide significant support for each project. The diabetes project has been managed by a full-time master's level project coordinator. This project has had a strong research emphasis and several presentations and papers have already been completed. Funding for this project has come from an internal discretionary research fund and a recently acquired external grant.

For all other projects, the CCE has used core resources for

■ assistance in development of the project;
■ development of the instruments used to collect the data;
■ creation of optically scannable data forms;
■ scanning and analysis of data;
■ tracking of patients who are enrolled in the outcomes study to ensure a complete data set; and
■ general technical supervision.

The CCE is now exploring ways to generate a medical record document from scanned outcomes data. They hope to minimize the need for dictating and/or writing notes and move the scanning process on site so the data are available for use during the office encounter. As this is accomplished, more of the history and physical exam data will be easily retrievable and analyzable for a variety of needs.

Thus far, all but one of the outcomes projects have been

conducted in the salaried Henry Ford Medical Group. The CCE is attempting to find ways to implement outcomes assessment in community hospitals that are part of the system and with private practitioners who are members of Independent Practice Association networks for the system HMO.

Cleveland Clinic Foundation, Office of Quality Management, Cleveland

The Cleveland Clinic Foundation is a large, multispecialty group practice comprising ambulatory care, a 1,000-bed acute-care hospital, and home health services. Outcomes assessment activity parallels the evolution, since 1990, of quality monitoring from a reactive, externally driven event to a proactive, comprehensive process with a research base. The Office of Quality Management was developed and a new department of Quality Research (QR) established. QR provides methods and measurement expertise to routine quality monitoring activities and manages and directs several outcomes assessment projects.

In 1991 three outcomes assessment projects were designed: total hip replacement, diabetes, and hypertension. Selection of conditions was based on the interest of key physicians and participation of the Cleveland Clinic Foundation in an AGPA consortium on pooling of outcomes data. Small pilot data samples were drawn with the initial aims of determining the feasibility of collecting outcomes data in a busy practice and the value of outcomes data to clinicians and administration. Health status and clinical indicators were collected longitudinally using available tools.

By 1992 requests for low back pain and cardiac valve projects generated a second set of projects. Currently, disease-specific health status indicators are being developed for cardiac valve surgery. All outcomes projects will have been evaluated by year-end 1993. It is expected some will become the framework for department-level quality monitoring and others will require more extensive research to refine disease-specific measures.

Initially, the outcomes assessment projects were implemented by the part-time activities of the QR director and a nurse epidemiologist. A staffing strategy has evolved for sharing staff, space, and equipment with the ongoing quality monitoring effort. This approach has been helpful in bridging the research and practice worlds. We all have come to represent "quality management" in the setting. The staff available for the outcomes projects now includes: the QR director (a PhD researcher), a statistician, a project manager (a PhD-candidate nurse), two data collectors, a data entry clerk, and a secretary.

BEFORE THE BEGINNING

To get started in outcomes assessment, a critical mass of leadership, financing, technical resources, and interest must be achieved. Rather than starting from scratch, it is usually preferable to build on existing resources and related activities within the organization. Even before a formal outcomes assessment initiative is launched, precursors can always be identified.

- There may be various clinical or health services research projects that incorporate patient outcomes into the study.
- A tumor registry continually monitors outcomes of a particular sort.
- Individuals with skills in project management, databases, and statistics may work for the organization.
- There may be a growing interest in an automated medical record.
- The local marketplace may be expressing increased demand for outcomes data.
- A visiting speaker may have stimulated interest in outcomes assessment among clinicians.

consensus

Precursors can become the raw materials for a broad-based outcomes assessment initiative. An early inventory of potential resources and advocates will help get things moving more quickly.

THE CATALYST

Organizational commitment is needed to get an outcomes effort underway. Someone (preferably more than one individual) within the organization needs to be a catalyst for change. The catalyst's role is to lead the charge for outcomes assessment and to coalesce the organizational resources needed to conduct a successful outcomes demonstration project. The catalytic reaction may be dramatic; more often it is a gradual transformation.

Identifying the Catalyst

One or more potential catalysts may emerge when inventorying organizational resources "before the beginning." The higher the catalyst's position in the organization, the more likely it is that an outcomes assessment effort will get underway. Someone in a position of influence is best able to assemble the key elements needed to start a project and to instill the outcomes vision among potential participants.

Although leadership from the top is important, the mission of outcomes assessment must not be perceived by clinicians as a management tool imposed upon them by the administration. Breadth of support is essential if the outcomes initiative is to advance beyond very early piloting.

consensus

Early strong leadership from top management is important and should be cultivated. However, a successful program can be developed even if the CEO never becomes a full-scale champion for outcomes assessment. To get underway, an outcomes initiative must have certain key elements in place:

- A few committed clinicians;
- Enough resources to conduct a pilot project;
- Access to the core technical skills needed in running the project; and
- At least a moderate level of support and interest from top management.

A catalyst with vision, energy, and influence can get the chemical reaction started.

Reason for Catalyst's Buy-In

Potential catalysts are motivated by a variety of factors, including

- purchaser demand;
- quality improvement; and
- scientific interest.

For most of our organizations, the most highly placed catalysts of outcomes assessment were motivated to act in anticipation of perceived purchaser demand. There is increasing agreement that the health care system needs to demonstrate the value of its services by means of outcomes data. This convergence of opinion has coalesced into explicit demand for outcomes data in only a few markets. Clinical executives who advocate outcomes assessment are "reading the tea leaves," positioning themselves for future trends in the marketplace.

CQI has been another key motivator for highly placed administrators to become catalysts for outcomes assessment. The CQI and outcomes assessment "movements" are philosophically compatible.

- Both define quality from the perspective of the patient.
- Both rely on clinicians' internal motivation to improve the quality of care.
- Both emphasize the need to measure the impact of change.

Clinician catalysts are more often drawn by the scientific underpinnings of outcomes assessment. Some want to add health status indicators to their ongoing research. Others want to start publishing in professional journals or making presentations at conferences. Still others simply want to know in quantitative terms how their patients are responding to care.

consensus

Customer demand, CQI, and science, especially in combination, are powerful incentives for launching an outcomes assessment effort. Purchasers can instill the sense of urgency needed to get a new activity going. Top management's commitment to CQI can build a pathway for integrating outcomes assessment into routine operations. Appealing to clinicians' scientific curiosity can prevent an outcomes assessment initiative from being perceived as an externally imposed management tool.

Shaping the Catalyst's Expectations

Probably the biggest payoff for outcomes assessment is in managing outcomes; that is, in improving the processes of care to generate better outcomes. However, the early stages of implementation demand almost exclusive attention to the measurement and monitoring functions. Outcomes assessment catalysts may be at risk of overselling the concept and building unrealistic expectations for dramatic early benefits of the effort.

consensus

The catalyst should be encouraged to communicate
the vision as a long-term direction, toward which
programmatic efforts must be directed. It should be
made clear to all stakeholders (clinicians, administrators, purchasers) that the payoffs of outcomes assessment accrue over the long term. The outcomes
implementation team needs to work toward fulfilling
the catalyst's vision through appropriate project
design and roll out. The catalyst should be frequently
updated on program goals and progress.

Relation to Organizational Goals

The effort to design and implement an outcomes assessment
initiative is considerable, requiring cultural change within the
organization. If the effort fits well with the organization's goals
and directions, implementation of outcomes assessment should go
more smoothly and, possibly, more rapidly.

Optimally, outcomes assessment will be directly congruent
with the larger organization's goals. Congruence may be evi-
denced by references in the corporate mission statement to
demonstrating value, measuring outcomes of care, and continually improving the quality of care as indicated by outcomes. If this
outcomes-oriented philosophy permeates the organization, then
individual departments are also likely to express their mission and
goals in terms of quantifiable outcomes. The outcomes assessment
program thus becomes integral to achieving the overall corporate
mission.

A less integrative mission statement may call for the establishment of an outcomes project as part of a larger organizational
objective. For example, an outcomes center may be created as a
resource for health services research or marketing, or quality

assurance, or as a separate developmental project. The danger is that the outcomes initiative may become isolated, unable to fulfill its role as organizational change agent.

If the corporate mission lacks an outcomes orientation, this shortcoming should be targeted for change as soon as possible. The outcomes catalyst or program director should take steps to communicate the purpose of outcomes assessment and to see that it becomes incorporated into the corporate direction. It is not necessary that these steps be completed before work begins. In fact, early results may help convince organizational leaders of the strategic importance of outcomes assessment.

consensus

> The catalyst and outcomes director should communicate to corporate planners the larger vision: that outcomes assessment can help establish an empirical basis for clinical decision making, patterns of care, and quality improvement. Given the limited state of the art in outcomes methodology, fulfillment of this vision will most likely occur incrementally, through pilot projects. Organizationwide integration of the outcomes assessment function is a long-term objective, achieved through phases of more limited implementation.

STRATEGIC PLANNING

Rosabeth Moss Kanter defines strategic planning as the "deliberate and conscious articulation of a direction."[*] Outcomes assessment points in a direction: toward equipping clinicians with the skills

---

[*] Kanter RM: *The Change Masters: Innovation and Entrepreneurship in the American Corporation.* New York: Simon & Schuster, 1983, p 294.

and information to evaluate and improve their own effectiveness; toward establishing a more informed and sophisticated dialogue among clinicians, administrators, and purchasers; and toward equipping patients with the knowledge to make truly informed decisions about their own care.

The big question is how to get the organization's early forays into outcomes assessment moving in the right direction. Should there be a top-down strategy for achieving organizationwide commitment to outcomes assessment? Or should progress take a more opportunistic course, building on the expressed interest of early adopters of the outcome vision among the clinicians?

Most of our sites have benefited from the advocacy of a highly placed catalyst in getting an outcomes initiative underway. However, in actually planning the work, our experience to date more closely approximates the bottom-up, opportunistic model. Although we are not sure whether this approach is either optimal or inevitable, there are some justifications:

- Clinician advocacy and participation is essential to the success of any outcomes project.
- Clinicians display a general mistrust of most top-down organizational initiatives.
- Attempts to impose a top-down strategy are apt to be perceived as an attempt to constrain clinicians' autonomy and judge their performance in a potentially punitive fashion.

Although outcomes projects tend to be launched from the bottom up, there will likely be a gradual infusion of top-down elements. For example, new projects may be begun only if they are perceived as a high priority on the basis of cost or prevalence. Clinicians from various outcomes projects may begin to meet together to discuss shared interests. Attention may shift to building an information systems infrastructure to support all outcomes projects.

consensus

It is desirable to plan the type of outcomes assessment initiative that can permeate the organization. This means planning a *process* of risk taking, problem solving, and unfolding. In the beginning there appears to be an advantage for the outcomes group to be perceived as somewhat of a guerrilla operation: supportive of grass-roots interest by the clinicians, not corrupted by a top-down institutional agenda. As early efforts take root, more strategic considerations will begin to unfold almost spontaneously.

FUNCTION WITHIN THE ORGANIZATION

An outcomes assessment program may consist of a single project, or it may encompass a wide array of activities. Its staff may be either the part-time activities of one person or a centralized group. In either event, the outcomes initiative needs to establish an identity. We identified four models by which an outcomes assessment program can define itself vis-à-vis the larger organization:

1. As an *operating division*. The outcomes program would function as a separate business unit, pursuing its own agenda in semiautonomy from the rest of the organization.
2. As a *service bureau*. The program would serve as staff support, performing functions needed by other operating divisions of the organization.
3. As an *internal consulting firm*. The program would provide technical expertise to other divisions on a per-project basis.
4. As a *leadership group*. The program would advocate a mission and promote culture change throughout the organization.

consensus

All of these models are valuable, and the outcomes assessment group will play each role at one time or another. However, it is particularly important that the outcomes assessment team be regarded as a combined internal consultant and leader. The role of change agent is best implemented by being responsive to internal customers and by doing technically proficient work on their behalf.

PLACEMENT IN THE ORGANIZATION

Early Phases

First generation outcomes assessment programs have developed in a variety of organizational niches. In some instances the outcomes work was begun within an existing department, typically an internal research group or a specific clinical specialty department. At other sites the work was initiated anew, with dedicated staff established in a separate department of the organization. We expect the next wave of sites to emerge in various ways.

There are several types of operating divisions that can serve as a home for outcomes assessment: quality assurance, CQI, health services research, information systems, or medical records. Establishing an outcomes assessment effort within an existing operating entity is a mixed blessing.

On a positive note, integration within the larger health care organization is compatible with the overall mission of outcomes assessment. Pragmatically, it may be possible to piggyback outcomes activities with related ongoing work. Outcomes work may also be buffered somewhat from political and financial maneuvering by being part of an established organizational unit.

On the other hand, outcomes assessment's broader vision and role as change agent may be compromised by having to fulfill other operational roles. In some instances we have met with enthusiasm from clinicians precisely because the outcomes group represents an alternative to more mainstream administrative programs. There may, however, be resistance from those established activities that perceive a threat in the increased attention directed toward outcomes assessment.

The meta-issue of "research versus operations" arises in considering organizational placement. If outcomes assessment is located in a research area on the organizational chart, it may be subject to some unwanted baggage: requirements to submit each project to the internal review board, having its agenda perceived as a series of projects rather than a coherent whole, and/or not being able to obtain adequate central staffing to support ongoing outcome monitoring. On the other hand, if the outcomes group is located in an operational area, it may face the danger of unrealistic expectations regarding pace of implementation.

consensus

> The goal is to get started: Be opportunistic. An established organizational unit can serve as an incubator for the new outcomes assessment initiative. Wherever the outcomes effort is housed, it should focus on pursuing the larger mission and nurturing informal communication networks across structural boundaries.

Transition

As the outcomes group becomes established, the larger organization tends to explore the possibilities of merging outcomes assessment with quality assurance, quality improvement, and utilization review or into a larger clinical information systems department. We regard this as a potential problem.

It is true that these programs share a common function: obtaining, interpreting, and feeding back information that helps clinicians examine their performance. An amalgamated department would conceivably include clinical and claims-based information systems, data management, and statistical expertise. Economies of scale should accrue from this sort of realignment. Outcomes assessment, however, has a mission that extends beyond the information systems and the data. In its purest form, outcomes assessment embodies an interpretive, responsive, interactive change-agent orientation.

In establishing an outcomes assessment effort, organizational placement should support the mission, roles, and strategy. We envision three distinct phases of organizational placement for an outcomes group:

1. **Guerrilla.** To encourage bottom-up support and rapid response to opportunities, the early outcomes initiative should be loosely linked to the preexisting bureaucracy.

2. **Coordinated infrastructure.** Many of the technical components of outcomes assessment—database construction, some data collection, data management, routine analyses—can be centralized in an expanded information systems group. The outcomes assessment team will concentrate on facilitating the *use* of outcomes data in understanding and improving care. Core activities will shift from measurement and monitoring to management: feedback, interpretation, linkage to clinical process, and education of clinicians in how to use quantitative information.

3. **Decentralization and integration.** Ultimately, outcomes assessment should become an aspect of the care process. The medical record will be structured and automated, supporting outcomes analyses. Clinicians will have the

ability to interpret statistical analyses. Reports and database searches will be available at the time of an encounter, supporting informed decision making by the clinician and the patient. In that future paradise, a separate outcomes group may no longer be necessary.

consensus

In the short term, an outcomes assessment group must involve itself in all phases of the work. In the long term, however, we see ourselves primarily as transformers of data into information, knowledge, and improved care. The *technology* of outcomes can be centralized into a larger organizational unit. However, the core mission remains the *management* of outcomes—establishing a quantitative basis for clinical care throughout the system. In planning for the long term, the technical functions should not be allowed to dominate the consultative and leadership roles.

ORGANIZATION OF THE OUTCOMES ASSESSMENT PROGRAM

The most important organizational issue facing an outcomes assessment effort is an internal one: How will the work get done? From small pilot projects to large integrated programs, the work of outcomes assessment must be managed and staffed.

Management

The overall director of the outcomes initiative should be identified. This person should be a leader, upholding the ultimate mission of outcomes assessment and serving as the primary agent of organizational change. Key operational functions of the director are planning, integrating outcomes assessment with organizational strategy, and generally directing the program.

Staffing Requirements

The core functions of an outcomes assessment *program* are identical to those functions needed to conduct an outcomes assessment *project*. These functions are described in more detail in Chapter 2, Project Management. Briefly, the key roles are

- project design;
- project coordination;
- instrumentation;
- protocol specification;
- data collection;
- data entry;
- data quality control;
- data storage;
- data analysis;
- feedback and interpretation;
- linkage to clinical process; and
- education and training.

In addition to specific technical skills, outcomes assessment staff should possess a general research and development orientation. All members of the team should strive for excellence in communicating, organizing, problem solving, asking questions, listening, and innovating. All should embody the change-agent role: embracing and inducing change, tolerating ambiguity, and championing the big ideas.

consensus

Technical proficiency is required. However, cheerleader/diplomat/counselor/detective skills are extremely important among outcome team members.

Central Staff

The size of the staff should match the size of the program, defined primarily in terms of the number and scope of projects underway. A small program may have a single individual fulfilling several roles, with some of the highly specialized functions being outsourced. A large program may devote one or more full-time employees to each core function.

Each of the network sites has assembled a central outcomes staff, capable in the aggregate of performing all the necessary outcomes assessment functions. Alternatively, an organization may be able to piece together the necessary technical staff from various departments (for example, quality assurance, clinical research, information systems).

To date, none of our sites has experienced a radical centralization of all measurement activities into one large department. Likewise, we have not participated in a radical decentralization, with outcomes assessment being fully integrated into the care system. Consequently, staffing requirements for these new phases are largely speculative.

consensus

In early phases the bulk of the outcomes assessment work is organized around achieving project-specific efficiency in measurement and monitoring: a core technical staff of one or more is needed. Over time the responsibility of the outcomes program will make a gradual transition to outcomes *management,* encouraging use of the data and analyses to change the way clinical care is delivered. A lean, high-level outcomes staff will focus on strategy, communication with information systems and clinical staff, and education and training. This high-level management group may or may not remain coupled with the technical staff responsible for measurement and monitoring.

Decentralized Functions

As our programs mature we are beginning to decentralize certain functions. Project-specific data collection and entry responsibilities are being shifted to the clinical departments. Project management may likewise become a clinical staff responsibility. We are equipping clinicians with the competencies needed to work comfortably with the data and analyses. Data quality and storage activities will ultimately be transferred to the information systems department. Even data analysis could conceivably move to an expanded information systems group.

The greater the decentralization of function, the better the possibility for clinician buy-in to outcomes assessment. However, a decentralization strategy brings with it a potential danger: diffusion of responsibility. How can the outcomes central staff manage functions over which they have no organizational authority?

consensus

There is a broad movement in health care toward organizational structures that are cross-functional, multidisciplinary, patient-centered and condition-centered, data driven, and quality improving. As a new entity unburdened by traditional organizational boundaries, the outcomes assessment program should model the new ways of organizing.

COMMUNICATION LINKS

Outcomes assessment is a developmental enterprise. Most health care organizations seem to be undergoing perpetual transition.

Consequently, we think it is unwise to spend too much time on structural issues affecting outcomes assessment. Functions and relationships are more important. To achieve culture change, the outcomes assessment team must build a network of like-minded individuals across departmental boundaries.

It is important to identify the individuals and groups whose buy-in is critical to organizational implementation. We have found it important to focus on leaders in the physician and nurse communities. Of particular value are the "champions"—present and potential users of outcomes data who strongly endorse the concept and who understand implementation issues. These individuals should be involved in strategic planning for outcomes activities, at least in an advisory capacity. They should also be encouraged to communicate the concept and strategy to their peers and subordinates throughout the organization.

consensus

As a new entity, the outcomes assessment team needs to identify friends and to avoid making enemies. Two-way communication is critical: asking for information, advice, and counsel, as well as informing about plans, approaches, and successes.

2
Project Management

In implementing outcomes assessment, the bulk of the work is concentrated in managing individual projects. This section describes a typical outcomes project, the sequence of activities that constitute a project, and the staffing and resources needed to accomplish the various activities.

A Case Study of an Outcome Project: Total Hip Replacement, Park Nicollet Medical Center (PNMC)

The first outcomes assessment project of PNMC's Outcomes Demonstration and Feasibility Project was for total hip replacement in the department of orthopedics. This surgical intervention was selected for reasons of both convenience and strategy. It was convenient because of the considerable interest expressed by the orthopedists in collecting long-term outcomes data. Strategically, the number of hip replacement surgeries was sufficiently small to allow for testing the feasibility of data collection, data management, analysis, and reporting. Hip replacement is also a high-cost and much-studied procedure.

The total hip replacement project was organized by the outcomes program director and the department chair. Meetings were held with all of the surgeons who perform this procedure to specify the purpose and scope of the project. Because this was our first initiative, its purpose remained vaguely defined: to collect longitudinal data on all patients having a total hip replacement performed by a PNMC orthopedist over a period of five to ten years. The long-term nature of the project was essential to the orthopedists' interest in the data collection. The nurse supervisor of the department served as the initial project contact.

As soon as the topic was selected, work began on development of outcomes questionnaires. The basic instruments used were the total hip replacement *TyPE* questionnaires for patients and clinicians, which are available from the Health Outcomes Institute (formerly InterStudy).* Some minor additions and format modifications were made in order to make the questionnaires easier to administer. Clinician forms were made as brief as possible, focusing on those data items that the doctor would typically collect during an encounter. Patient forms were made as self-explanatory as possible so that the staff time would be minimized during administration. This meant attaching an easy-to-understand cover letter, using a large print font, and using categorical responses for every item. To minimize staff burden, scannable forms were developed to allow rapid, accurate data entry.

The data collection intervals—preoperative, 3 months postop, 12 months postop, annually thereafter—were specified in the TyPE documentation and were adopted by the ortho group. The nurse supervisor communicated the data collection protocols as developed by the outcomes program director to the nursing staff. We developed an automated "tickler" and tracking system that staff could use to identify who needed to be contacted for follow-up questionnaires during specific time intervals.

The nurse supervisor also implemented the initial data completeness checks. A first check ensured that the outcomes questionnaires were being completed by the patient. Eventually this

---

* InterStudy has compiled several instruments—collectively called *TyPEs* (Technology of Patient Experience)—for use in measuring outcomes. See page 118 for more information on TyPE questionnaires.

function was performed in real time, just after the patient returned the questionnaire to the office staff person. A second completeness check involved identifying what percentage of all patients eligible for participation in the project were actually being enrolled. This process involved comparing the names of patients captured on the outcomes data forms with the names on the surgery schedule. These activities were shifted to a project coordinator on the outcomes project staff at approximately the beginning of year two of data collection.

One major activity of the outcomes work at PNMC was to create a database that could be used for outcomes data from any department. At first, data were entered into this system manually, performed centrally by the project coordinator. The subsequent development of scannable forms allowed the data entry function to be transferred back to orthopedics department staff. The project coordinator continued to perform data completeness checks as well as verification of the accuracy of data entry.

Analysis of the patient and physician data also began during the second year and consisted primarily of descriptive statistics. These were summarized into a quarterly report to the physicians by the project analyst on the outcomes project staff. Initially, reports were presented to the physicians in the context of a special meeting conducted by the outcomes staff. Physicians reviewed the results and were asked to comment on any findings that appeared unexpected or anomalous.

In one of these physician reviews, the orthopedists defined a key component in the care process that they perceived as causing undesired variation in outcomes. A corresponding plan for process improvement was subsequently developed. It remains somewhat unclear how the improvement plan will be implemented by the department because of the lack of an identified orthopedics staff member with that responsibility.

STEPS IN IMPLEMENTING AN OUTCOMES PROJECT

An outcomes assessment project can be characterized in terms of a series of steps to be accomplished.

1. Make a commitment to begin.
   a. Identify a condition or procedure to investigate;
   b. Assemble a project team; and
   c. Name a project coordinator.
2. Design the project.
   a. Define the purpose of the project;
   b. Define the scope of the project;
   c. Develop the measurement instruments to be used; and
   d. Establish a logistical protocol for data collection.
3. Manage the data.
   a. Collect the data;
   b. Enter the data into a database;
   c. Maintain quality control over the data; and
   d. Store the data.
4. Use the data.
   a. Analyze the data;
   b. Provide feedback and interpretation to clinicians; and
   c. Link outcomes to the clinical process.

Each of these steps is discussed in greater detail in the following section.

COMMITMENT TO BEGIN

Identifying a Condition or Procedure

The first step in a new outcomes project is to decide which condition or procedure to study. A top-down strategic approach may use specific criteria for selecting project topics; for example, the ten costliest conditions or the top five procedures by volume. In our experience a new project is initiated largely through discussions between the director of the outcomes assessment effort and an interested clinician.

Some conditions and procedures are more difficult than others to measure and to monitor. The degree of difficulty is a function of a number of factors, including

- potential controversy surrounding the project;
- organizational complexity;
- objectives to be achieved;
- types of patients;
- number of patients;
- availability of measurement tools; and
- logistical complexity.

consensus

All outcomes assessment projects are difficult. Start with the comparatively easier ones, then move to the more difficult ones after accruing some experience.

Some potential projects are more controversial than others, for example:

- There may be significant disagreements about how best to treat a particular condition;
- Clinicians may overtly disagree about what types of outcomes (for example, physiology, functional status) are most important; and
- A potential project may require close cooperation between feuding departments.

consensus

Avoid controversy wherever possible. There are enough obstacles to successful implementation without having to contend with political disputes.

Assembling a Team

Each of our sites uses the same basic model for project management. The clinicians "own" the project, and the outcomes staff provides consulting and necessary management services for the project.

A project team sets the goals of the project and monitors progress. The project's earliest course of development is usually set by the outcomes program director and the clinician project champion. But a more formal team should be configured as early as possible. Its core consists of those clinicians who are particularly interested in the project and a project coordinator. However, all clinicians whose patients will be included in data collection should be given an opportunity to participate. Specialists in the technology of outcomes assessment should be called in as needed.

consensus

Again, we recommend starting with easier projects. It is easier to assemble an effective project team when all participating clinicians come from the same department. For example, assessing the outcomes of hip replacement surgery involves mainly orthopedists. In contrast, treatment of low back pain typically covers various specialties.

The Project Coordinator

The project coordinator brings together all the skills and resources needed to carry out a project. The coordinator thus serves as both a task manager and a liaison between clinicians and clinical staff and the outcomes assessment technical staff. The person serving in this role may come from either the central outcomes assessment staff or a clinical department.

Perhaps to a greater extent than other technical specialists in outcomes assessment, a project coordinator should possess the general competencies of a change agent in communicating, problem solving, innovating, and championing the larger agenda. Especially important are interpersonal communication skills. Contact with individuals throughout the institution often requires considerable sensitivity to competing professional and personal agendas, as well as an ability to avert possible conflicts in a nonadversarial manner. The role is a challenging one; the coordinator has many of the responsibilities of a manager, but may not have the corresponding authority over the project team members.

consensus

One individual can reasonably coordinate from one to five projects, depending on the size, scope, and phase of the projects. The beginning of a project requires concentrated effort in design, organization, and buy-in. As a project matures to a maintenance stage, less active intervention, and consequently less time, is demanded of the project coordinator.

DESIGN

The design of an outcomes assessment project consists of

- a statement of purpose;
- the scope of the data capture activity;
- instruments for measuring outcomes and other relevant constructs;
- the logistics of collecting the data; and
- data analysis requirements.

Purpose

The primary purpose underlying most pilot projects is feasibility: Can we collect data routinely and efficiently on all eligible patients? It is important for everyone, including funders and clinicians, to understand the importance of high-quality data in achieving the larger vision of outcomes assessment.

Ultimately, an outcomes assessment project should be designed to achieve some purpose within the health care system. Agreeing on this higher-order purpose for an outcomes project is essential, yet surprisingly difficult. Some possibilities include

- comparing one treatment with another for effectiveness in the routine treatment of a particular condition;
- describing in measurable terms the typical course of a chronic disease;
- using variations in outcome to identify opportunities for improving clinical process; and
- developing decision support programs for use with individual patients when choosing among alternative treatment options.

Each participant in the project comes to the table with an agenda. One may be interested in publishable clinical research, another in marketing the department's excellence, a third in continuous quality improvement. To some extent the same project can fulfill multiple purposes. However, trying to be too broad in focus may compromise the quality of the project.

consensus

Be conservative in expectations. Achieving good implementation logistics—collecting the data on the right patients at the right times—is a major challenge and should be an objective of every project. In addition, a primary use of the data should be specified and agreed to by everyone involved in the project. At least initially, simply trying to describe the outcomes of care in quantitative terms is an ambitious undertaking. Other uses of the data (such as hypothesis testing

and predictive modeling) should be attempted only
after the logistical and descriptive work has succeeded.

Scope

The project scope defines the criteria for including patients in the
data collection effort. Two key questions must be addressed.

1. What kinds of patients will be included in the project? Most
   projects focus on a specific diagnosis or procedure. However, it is certainly possible to devise outcome projects that
   cover a number of related diagnoses.

consensus

Begin by limiting the project to a single diagnosis or
procedure. Looking simultaneously at multiple
diagnoses adds both to the size of the project (more
patients to manage logistically) and to its complexity
(instrument design and analysis).

2. How many patients will be included in the project? Will
   data be collected on all patients seen by all clinicians in the
   organization? Or will there be a predetermined sample size
   based on power calculations?

consensus

Begin with a small pilot project, involving a small
number of patients identified over a short time
interval. Invariably the protocol will need some
revision, which can then be made without compromising the larger project. Success in the pilot can
build confidence; failure can be diagnosed and
corrected in a nonthreatening context.

Instruments

Instruments are needed for measuring the various constructs to be assessed in the project. A single outcomes assessment project may include instruments for identifying

- diagnosis;
- demographics;
- clinical laboratory values (for example, blood gases);
- signs and symptoms (for example, chest pain);
- functional status (for example, ability to climb a flight of stairs); and
- treatment process.

Most outcomes assessment projects rely heavily on patient self-report questionnaires for demographics, functional status, and symptoms. Structured clinical data forms are used for diagnosis, lab value readings, and treatment specifications. The clinicians themselves may complete the forms, or the data may be captured via retrospective chart review.

How does an outcomes project obtain the appropriate measurement instruments? One option is to use existing instruments. The task of selecting instruments requires close liaison with the clinicians to identify what constructs need to be measured. An appropriate measurement tool may be identified through a search of the clinical literature, discussion with clinicians, or networking with other outcomes assessment initiatives. In selecting an existing instrument it is important to evaluate its statistical reliability and validity and its appropriateness for the specific project.

An alternative approach is to design instruments from scratch: decide what needs to be measured; devise a valid and practical measurement tool; and continually refine the tool based on feedback from patients, clinicians, project administrators, and biostatisticians. The person charged with developing outcomes instruments should have a background in psychometrics and statistics and should be able to work with clinicians in defining important constructs.

consensus

Seek instruments that are brief and easy to administer. Start with existing instruments wherever possible. However, we have almost always found it necessary to adapt instruments to the needs of the specific project. Until a battery of agreed-upon tools is available, an outcomes initiative should seek technical expertise in instrumentation. Unless a site anticipates running a large number of outcomes projects, this expertise is probably best secured from a consultant.

Logistics

Once the instruments have been gathered, methods must be defined for collecting the data from patients, clinicians, and/or medical records. Issues to be considered include the following:

- When will the data be collected (before and after initiation of a new treatment, immediately prior to an encounter)?
- How often will data be collected (every office visit, once per year)?
- Where will data be collected (at the physician's office, at the patient's home)?
- Who will collect the data (patient self-administered questionnaire, chart review by a technician)?

Designing an effective outcomes monitoring protocol requires a delicate balance between methodological rigor and pragmatics. The outcomes assessment activity must be adapted to fit the work flow and organization of the clinical care setting, not vice versa. The design team should work closely with clinicians and/or administrative support staff to engineer an efficient protocol that minimizes disruption to the ongoing care delivery processes.

consensus

Begin with logistical simplicity. For example, don't start with a protocol that requires several departments' cooperation in getting the data collected. Minimize the burden of data collection on clinicians by asking patients to report directly on their own symptoms and functional status, on patient care flow by collecting patient follow-up data by mail rather than scheduling an unnecessary extra visit to the clinician's office, and on patients by not requiring emergency patients to complete questionnaires.

DATA MANAGEMENT

Data Collection

Data management is concerned with how to obtain complete and accurate data according to the protocol specifications. The design specifies when, how often, where, and from whom data will be collected. At each of our sites, the biggest challenge and greatest amount of effort go into achieving efficient data collection.

The mechanics of data collection vary along the following key dimensions.

Patient Data

1. **During an encounter**. Many protocols specify that at least some patient data be collected at an encounter; for example, at the patient's first visit to the physician, at a key decision point in the treatment of a chronic condition, or immediately prior to surgery. It is far easier to collect encounter data if the clinical staff, rather than the central outcomes staff, are responsible for identifying eligible patients, distributing questionnaires, and ensuring proper comple-

tion of the forms. As previously noted, all our sites rely heavily on patient self-administration of questionnaires. Some clinicians opt to administer the questionnaires in a structured interview format. Obviously this method is more labor intensive. However, to the extent that the outcomes questionnaires can be incorporated into the clinician's routine patient work-up, the structured interview may actually increase the efficiency of data capture.

2. **By mail.** A protocol may call for patient data to be collected at particular time intervals (for example, post-surgical follow-up, periodic monitoring of patients with a chronic condition). A mail-out/mail-back strategy may work for this sort of protocol. In our sites, technicians from the central outcomes staff coordinate data collection by mail.

Clinician Data

In some sites the clinical form is completed by the clinician or staff during or immediately after an encounter. This option works particularly well if the clinicians agree to use the structured data forms to replace portions of the medical record. An alternative is to rely on retrospective chart review, which is acceptable only if the clinician does not intend to use the outcomes data during the encounter and if the necessary data can be reliably retrieved from the medical record.

Outcomes assessment requires repeated measures for each patient. A timely and effective tickler system is needed to trigger the data collection cycle at the appropriate times, as specified by the project protocols. Some sites use a manual log; others have an automated reminder system. At a minimum, the tickler should identify which data forms should be collected, from whom, and when. It should also identify cases in which scheduled forms have not yet been completed so that a follow-up contact may be initiated.

consensus

It is optimal if the clinicians and their staff assume
ownership of the data collection process. For this to
occur they must value the information to be obtained.
As early in the project as possible, involve the clinicians and their staff in modifying instruments and
designing protocols that enhance rather than burden
the care process.

Data Entry

Once collected, the data must be entered into a database. There are
three primary decisions to be made with respect to data entry.
First, is it important that data be entered in real time, or can entry
be delayed? Second, will data entry be manual or automated?
Third, who should be responsible for performing the data entry
function?

Real Time or Batch?

It is easier to delay data entry until several completed forms can be
entered at the same time. We have found that batch data entry is
most efficient when centralized in the outcomes assessment unit.
However, there may be reasons why data should be entered
immediately after the form is completed. The provider may, for
example, wish to compare the patient's current health status with
last month's score or with similar patients during the encounter. If
real-time feedback is required, data entry will almost certainly
need to take place in the clinical unit. The design of the project
and anticipated uses of the data will dictate whether the logistically easier batch method can be used.

Manual or Automated?

Manual data entry is largely a clerical function that can be performed successfully with minimal training. Automated data entry
is also possible. Scanners, or optical mark readers, are used at some
sites, and there has been discussion of using touch screen technol-

ogy or computer-assisted telephone interviewing systems. Automated methods are more expensive to build and install than
manual methods, but they can achieve significant economies in
the long term. They should be considered if the organization
anticipates a large volume of data. Automated data entry is
probably the preferred option if real-time feedback of data analysis
is needed.

Who Is Responsible?

If the clinicians need real-time data entry during the encounter,
the clinical department will need to assume responsibility for data
entry. The central outcomes staff should provide technical support
to the clinical staff in making this transition to decentralized data
entry. If a feedback delay is acceptable (for example, when aggregate rather than patient-specific results are of prime concern), it is
probably easier for the outcomes group to handle the task, either
with in-house staff or through an external data entry contractor.

Data Quality Control

Data must be checked for completeness, accuracy, and compliance
with protocols. This function should be performed at several steps
in the data management process.

1. Missing or faulty data should be identified at the time of
   data collection, when the data source (that is, the patient or
   provider) is available to correct the problem.
2. Incomplete or seriously flawed data forms should also be
   identified at the time of data entry.
3. Some sites use double entry to ensure accuracy, that is, two
   coders independently enter data from the same form, then
   look for discrepancies.
4. The database should be programmed to check for values
   that are out of range, illogical, or missing before storing the
   information permanently in the database.

5. The surgery or clinic schedule and/or the claims database should be reviewed frequently to determine that all eligible patients have been included in the project.

The larger and more complex the project, the greater the difficulty in maintaining data quality. The quality control function is a valuable source of information for continually improving the overall data management function. Quality control summary reports should be provided to the project coordinator at timely intervals.

Standards for data quality and methods for quality control should be established by someone with expertise in database management and research methodology. Monitoring the data for quality failures is a clerical function, much of which can be automated and/or assigned to data entry personnel. Error correction requires problem-solving skills as well as the ability to work with individuals throughout the sequence of data collection and entry activities.

Data Storage

Ensuring data integrity, merging and downloading files, managing access and confidentiality, and maintaining hardware and software are traditional information systems activities. To date, all network sites have accomplished this function for outcomes data within the outcomes assessment unit. Ultimately this role will probably be filled by the institution's information systems department.

USE OF DATA

Data Analysis

Outcomes data must be scored and analyzed to achieve the purposes of the project.

Analyses may be

- aggregate or patient specific;
- database queries or more complex statistical analyses; or
- routine reports or special studies.

The data analyst must understand the nature of each outcomes project, the strengths and weaknesses of the data, the perspectives of the clinicians and administrators, and the potential uses of the data. Knowledge of statistics is needed, including experience with multivariate methods, repeated measures, and statistical quality control techniques. Sites that do not have in-house access to sufficient analytical expertise should seek a statistical consultant. If several projects are anticipated, it will probably be necessary to hire a data analyst.

Feedback and Interpretation

Data analysis requires statistical expertise; interpretation of findings requires clinical expertise. It should be acknowledged, however, that most clinicians and administrators are not adept at interpreting statistical information. Analyses must be presented in ways that project participants can understand and use. Some sites generate a set of standard reports; others do not. In either event, someone from the outcomes technical staff should regularly discuss results with the clinicians. Communication and explanatory skills are required, as well as a basic understanding of the statistics involved.

Linking Outcome to Process

It is important that the outcomes analyses be used in evaluating and improving the effectiveness of the care process. This function resides largely with the clinicians. However, linking outcome information to clinical processes is made much more straightforward if the instruments, analyses, and feedback mechanisms are designed with this purpose in mind.

consensus

A long-term goal of outcomes assessment is to give clinicians direct access to usable quantitative information. In these early evolutionary stages of outcomes methodology, the transformation from raw outcomes data to useful information demands a considerable degree of exploratory statistical work and frequent data interpretation sessions with the clinicians.

To achieve true efficiency and integration with the care process, it is important that most statistical analyses become standardized, routinized, and possibly automated. At the same time, clinicians must be taught how to interpret these analyses and to use them in redesigning the care process. Outcomes assessment sites should work together toward increased standardization of analysis and feedback strategies.

DATABASE

Every outcomes project needs a database for entering, storing, editing, and querying the outcomes data and preparing the data for statistical analysis.

Key Design Features

A computer database should be designed to fit the character of the data being collected, the mechanisms for entering data, and the likely reporting and extraction requirements. Computer professionals with an understanding of clinical data, research, and time-oriented data can be valuable in designing the database. They should be brought in as soon as rough instrument forms and data collection protocols are available.

The outcomes database structure should

- be relational in structure;
- support easy querying and sorting, eventually enabling clinicians to interact directly with the data;
- be flexible enough to be changed inexpensively as demands on the system change (for example, modifications to data fields, patient types, measurement intervals);
- be easily adapted to new projects; and
- have interfaces appropriate to all the likely users (patients, office staff, nurses, physicians, data entry clerks, researchers, and so forth).

consensus

The database should play a supporting role in outcomes assessment. Plan the data function on paper: what the questionnaires will look like, who will enter data, how data will be entered (that is, manually or via scanner), who will need to interact with the database, how data will be analyzed, what sorts of reports will be generated, and so forth. Build or buy the database that best supports the plan; do not build the plan around the database.

Stand-Alone or Integrated Database?

In designing a database, the biggest decision is whether to build a stand-alone outcomes database system, or to build outcomes capabilities into a general-purpose, centralized information system.

- **Stand-alone system.** All network sites started with a dedicated outcomes assessment database. In each case the system was built using a third-generation database language and implemented on a personal computer. Some sites used in-house programmers, others contracted out the work. No one used a ready-made system, since at the time there were no off-the-shelf products available. We expect that, at least in the near future, considerable customization will continue to be necessary.

■ **Centralized information system.** Outcomes data should ultimately become incorporated into the institutions' central information system. In most cases the core system is designed primarily to facilitate financial transactions; in other cases there may be a computerized medical record. To ensure that outcomes assessment needs are served, the outcomes staff should seek to participate actively in institutionwide information systems planning. Later transition to the larger system can be facilitated by building basic compatibility into the data structures; for example, by using the patient's medical record number as the patient identifier in the outcomes database.

Data Links

A health outcomes database includes a core set of data: patient identifiers, demographics, health status, symptoms, and clinical indicators. This core data set has typically been compiled anew: Outcomes data collection forms are designed, clinicians and patients complete the forms, and someone enters the data into a stand-alone database. However, there are existing data sets that can be found in other information systems within the organization. These databases often include data on

- cost/charges;
- patient satisfaction;
- utilization;
- process of care;
- demographics;
- comorbidities;
- mortality;

- major morbidity;
- registries; and
- case-mix or severity indexing.

Links to existing data sets can be extremely valuable to an outcomes assessment initiative.

1. An efficient implementation of outcomes assessment should avoid redundancy in data collection. If an existing database already contains reliable outcomes data and is readily retrievable at low cost, it is better to reuse the existing data than to collect it again.

2. The outcomes group should avoid the embarrassment or harm of asking questions to which they should already know the answers. For example, suppose a patient scheduled to complete a follow-up questionnaire died three months ago. Is there some way to tap into organizational information about patient deaths before mailing the questionnaire?

3. There may be important data questions that can be answered only by having access to other sorts of data. For example, the clinicians may want to know the relationship between health status improvement and patient satisfaction.

Data linkages depend on both organizational and technological factors.

- **Organizational linkages.** In gaining access to other data sets, the outcomes assessment team may benefit from building direct relationships with other departments. For example, if an outcomes assessment program is housed jointly with the quality assurance department, it will have easier access to data on utilization, mortality, and morbidity. On the other hand, the gain in data access may be offset by increased managerial complexity. There is also the danger of compromising working relations with the clinical departments, who are the ultimate customers of outcomes assessment.

consensus

In gaining access to relevant databases, placement within the organizational structure is less important than informal communication networks. The outcomes director must learn what data are available, who controls them, how to obtain them, and how to interpret them.

■ **Technological linkages.** There are four levels of complexity, listed below, in linking databases. The more strategic the implementation, the greater the justification for pursuing a complex linking method.

1. Obtain a hard copy of data, enter it manually into a separate database, then merge data into an analysis file.
2. Download relevant pieces of other databases electronically, then merge into an analysis file.
3. Build on-line links with other databases.
4. Build a massive relational database that includes all the data sets. This is the centralized information system option discussed on page 76.

consensus

Start with the easier linking technologies until you are confident of your long-term data needs. This confidence is usually built up after a few projects are well underway.

3
Financing

Organizing and administering an outcomes assessment effort requires a significant financial outlay. Costs depend both on the phase of implementation and on the anticipated scale of implementation. Sources of funding may be internal or external, in cash or in-kind, programmatic or project specific. Cost justification should be tied to organizational objectives, yet realistic in light of the developmental nature of outcomes assessment.

COST CATEGORIES

There are three general categories of costs involved in managing an outcomes assessment program: start-up, technology development, and ongoing operations. The manager of the outcomes effort should establish a budgeting and cost tracking mechanism based on these three categories.

Start-Up Costs

Putting an outcomes assessment program in place requires planning. Ideally an outcomes manager will already be in place to coordinate the planning effort. Key personnel in other departments will also need to be involved. Initial strategic planning may be aided by hiring consultants, attending selected seminars, and conducting on-site visits to established outcomes assessment programs. Once a strategic plan has been developed, core staff must be put in place (through hiring or contracting) and trained.

Technology Development

A technological infrastructure must be established. Technology may be bought off the shelf, customized, or built from scratch. Components include

- measurement instruments;
- database management system (hardware, software);
- data capture methods and interfaces;
- statistical analysis plans; and
- data reporting formats.

Ongoing Operations

Once the core staff and technology are in place, there are ongoing costs associated with outcomes assessment implementation. These are the costs associated with project management, including

- project design;
- project coordination;
- data collection;
- data entry;
- data quality control;
- data analysis; and
- feedback.

APPROPRIATE ALLOCATION OF COSTS

Costs should be appropriately allocated among the three cost categories in order to avoid two misinterpretations. First, lumping all start-up and development costs into an initial demonstration project may make outcomes assessment appear overly expensive. It is probably more appropriate to amortize these developmental costs over a longer time frame, spread across all subsequent outcomes projects that benefit from the initial investment.

Second, appropriate cost allocation also prevents start-up programs from the opposite misinterpretation of other programs' experiences; that is, of underestimating the cost of implementing an outcomes assessment project. Organizations planning an outcomes initiative should be cautious in basing cost estimates on the operating budgets of relatively mature outcomes assessment programs, without taking into account the previously incurred fixed expenses.

consensus

In its early implementation, outcomes assessment is a research and development activity. Start-up and technology development should be regarded not merely as "sunk costs" but as an investment in the organization. Generally speaking, the greater the up-front investment in planning and infrastructure for outcomes assessment, the lower the operating expenses later on.

Costs incurred outside of the outcomes core staff must also be considered. Clinicians and their support personnel may invest significant amounts of time in various aspects of outcomes assessment work. A decision should be made whether to assign these costs to the outcomes budget or to the clinical budget; this issue is addressed again in "Sources of Financing" (see page 84).

consensus

Projects typically begin on the central outcomes assessment budget. As proof of concept is established, it becomes possible to allocate ongoing costs to clinical department budgets.

VARIABLES IN BUDGETING

Budgeting for each cost category depends on the anticipated scale of implementation, the state of the art, and synergies to be achieved by integrating outcomes assessment with related functions.

Scale of Implementation

If a large-scale implementation is anticipated, total fixed costs (start-up, technology development) will almost certainly be higher. However, if these costs are amortized appropriately, economies of large-scale implementation should result in lower per-project costs.

State of the Art

Methodologically, outcomes assessment is in an early development stage. Instrumentation is of mixed quality; off-the-shelf technology is limited to specific applications; there is no consensus on analysis and feedback strategy. In the long run, development and dissemination of outcomes assessment technology will reduce implementation costs. In the short run, however, the more new ground a specific project covers, the higher the associated cost of development. The decision to proceed depends in part on personnel skills available to the outcomes assessment initiative and on the strategic importance of the project.

consensus

Use existing technology if possible. It will not be perfect, but your innovations will not be either. Experience in using the tools will give you the best idea of how to modify them. To avoid reinventing the wheel, network with other outcomes programs or participate in an interinstitutional collaborative project.

Possible Synergies

The clinical and functional status data used in outcomes assessment are just the sort of information that should appear in a patient's record. Structured and/or computerized medical records can result in significant cost savings for an outcomes assessment program. Other possibilities for synergy and cost savings can usually be found if communication channels are operating effectively.

consensus

> The automated medical record is in its early stages at most sites. Linking the outcomes work to this sort of major investment certainly takes a long-term perspective. It is unlikely to result in short-term cost justifications for outcomes assessment expenses. Nonetheless, building synergies between outcomes assessment and the automated medical record is a worthwhile effort, and one we are actively pursuing at each of the network sites.

How Much to Budget?

Organizations that have already implemented an outcomes assessment program are the best source of information on costs. Health care administrators or outcomes assessment directors should visit these organizations for benchmarking purposes. Nonetheless, there will be wide variations in cost estimates, staffing levels, types of personnel, and salaries. As previously noted, there may also be hidden or unestimated costs associated with start-up efforts; these should be explored.

SOURCES OF FINANCING

External Funding

Possible external funding sources for outcomes assessment are identified below *(followed by network consensus observations).*

- Research grant "piggybacking." Getting outcomes assessment activities incorporated into larger research or measurement activities, for example, external research grants, drug trials, nursing department program evaluations, continuous quality improvement studies. *(This has been a successful strategy at times for most of the network programs.)*
- Unrestricted foundation grants. *(Unlikely.)*
- Foundation project-specific grants. *(This is a good source, but beware of compromising the overall outcomes mission for the sake of fundable project-specific objectives.)*
- Government research agencies, for example, Agency for Health Care Policy Research (AHCPR), National Institute of Health (NIH). *(To date these agencies have not supported ongoing outcomes assessment activities. Currently they are more responsive to studies of condition-specific clinical effectiveness and the validation of outcomes measurement instruments.)*
- Institutional fundraising by the health care organization. *(This is a strong possibility, especially if there is a senior physician champion for outcomes assessment able to assume leadership in the campaign.)*
- Drug or device trials. *(These projects are usually unsuited to the needs of the organization's outcomes assessment effort.)*
- Consulting revenues. *(The technical expertise of an outcomes assessment staff is a marketable resource. Again, there is the danger of diluting the outcomes mission within the outcomes group's home organization.)*
- Payers. *(We have experienced some success here. It might be worth trying to negotiate administrative trade-offs, that is,

*building an outcomes assessment program in exchange for
eliminating other payer burdens such as precertification or
utilization review.)*

If external funds are desired, the outcomes assessment director
should initiate early discussions with the potential funder about
proposed grant activities, time frame for implementation, and
funding required. The external funder will probably expect the
organization to demonstrate its commitment by putting up seed
money.

consensus

Outcomes assessment is R&D, not clinical research as
usually defined. Consequently, it has little access to
traditional research funding sources. As the outcomes
"movement" expands, external support for demonstration projects will be increasingly difficult to obtain.
If outside funds are secured, begin planning for the
loss of those funds and the transition to internal
funding.

Internal Funding

Sources of internal funds include

- organizational operating revenues *(ultimately the primary
  source of funding, and beginning to happen at some sites)*;
- special project set-aside funds *(a good source if the organization has such a fund)*;
- marketing *(may be appropriate for funding patient surveys)*;
- specific clinical programs *(an effective source where outcomes
  assessment is seen as a strategic advantage in the marketplace)*;
- research/innovation funds *(to evaluate or to cost-justify a new
  service or technology)*;
- registry, for example, tumor or heart *(to rework or to extend
  an existing registry)*; and

■ information services *(use information systems staff, equipment, or existing databases in the outcomes assessment effort).*

Project Specific, Programmatic, or Operational?

Outcomes assessment will fulfill its potential to the extent that it permeates the clinical care process. This model of implementation implies that a significant proportion of the outcome program's budget should come from general revenues.

None of the network programs began this way, but all have made some movement in this direction. We expect project funding to move through a series of four phases.

1. At start-up, the outcomes assessment work will be funded as a pilot. Funding will be obtained either for individual demonstration projects or possibly for a more comprehensive program on a time-limited basis.

2. Once proof of concept has been attained, the outcomes assessment effort will become a standing R&D center. It will have its own operating budget, financed largely from operating revenues, allocated on both a general and a project-specific basis.

3. At some point, outcomes assessment will have permeated clinical practice to the point that costs of implementation will be regarded as part of the cost of care delivery.

4. Outcomes assessment becomes invisible, seamlessly integrated into routine care delivery.

This funding sequence is likely to occur one project at a time. One project may be funded as a pilot, another as an ongoing special initiative, and a third as part of routine clinical care.

consensus

Pilot projects are extremely vulnerable to budget cuts. So is overhead, which is how the R&D function might be labeled during tough times. Until outcomes

assessment becomes integrated with clinical care, its
funding will remain tenuous.

Cash or In-Kind?

As outcomes assessment becomes integrated with clinical care,
more responsibilities devolve from the centralized outcome staff to
the clinical staff. Clinicians participate in planning meetings and
reviewing analyses. Administrative staff become responsible for
collecting data from patients. For real-time systems, data entry
may also be decentralized.

Should these activities be budgeted and funded by the outcomes assessment program, with compensation flowing back to
the clinical departments? Or should these activities be regarded
as in-kind support for outcomes assessment from the clinical
departments?

consensus

The outcomes assessment program should not
compensate clinicians for in-kind costs. Ownership of
outcomes assessment must ultimately reside in the
clinical area; payment is one of the best demonstra-
tions of ownership. However, it is likely that clinicians
will need to become convinced of the value of
outcomes assessment before being willing to absorb
significant expenses. Plan toward a funding transition
path: from pilot project, funded by the outcomes
assessment program, to self-funded clinical
operations.

Relationship with the Funders

The outcomes assessment director should understand the funder's
agenda and be prepared to justify planned uses of funds (for
example, selection of specific projects) in light of that agenda. This

is true whether the funder is internal or external to the organization. However, it should be made clear that primary responsibility for strategic planning of outcomes assessment resides with the outcomes assessment team, not with the funder.

The outcomes assessment manager should ensure that internal funders do not expect immediate returns to the bottom line from outcomes assessment activities. Advocates of outcomes assessment, especially purchasers and insurers, often regard cost savings as the major motivation for outcomes initiatives. Although this expectation may ultimately prove valid, we believe that other justifications should be made dominant. These are discussed in more detail in Chapter 7, Demonstrating Value.

4

Education, Training, and Awareness Raising

The leaders of outcomes assessment must make sure that all key parties become equipped to carry out the mission. There are three broad classes of information exchange that must be made effective if implementation is to succeed on a continuing basis.

1. **Education** implies the transfer of general competencies. To become educated is to learn how to think, ask questions, and adapt to changing circumstances.

2. **Training** is the transfer of very specific skills, to be applied in specific circumstances, so as to generate predictable results in performance.

3. **Awareness raising** is the nurturing of a general understanding of, and enthusiasm for, an idea.

There are three basic issues to be addressed in devising a formal communication strategy.

1. **Who** needs to know? This chapter is organized around learning needs for each of the various constituencies involved in outcomes assessment: central outcomes staff, clinicians, project support staff, administration, and the broader community.

2. **What** do they need to know? Different people need to learn different skills, competencies, and information. Special

needs for education, training, and public awareness are addressed.

3. **How** should the learning experience be conducted? A variety of formats is possible, including traditional lecture, apprenticeship, and on-the-job training. Different methods are appropriate for different constituencies and for the different types of knowledge to be conveyed.

To illustrate key ideas, we present some examples of learning activities conducted by St Vincent Hospital in Portland, a member of the Sisters of Providence Health System, Oregon, by the Cleveland Clinic Foundation, and by the Henry Ford Health System.

OUTCOMES ASSESSMENT CENTRAL STAFF

Central staff consists of the core team responsible for providing technical support to outcomes assessment projects throughout the organization. Included are technical experts and project coordinators.

Education

Each central staffer should already possess a set of specific professional capabilities that qualifies him or her to fulfill a designated job on the outcomes program. To function effectively as a team and an organizational resource, staff should acquire a shared conceptual and functional framework for outcomes assessment. Components of the shared knowledge base include answers to the following questions:

- What is an outcome?
- What is outcomes assessment?
- How are outcomes measured?
- How are outcomes analyzed?
- How are outcomes analyses used in clinical care?

Also needed is a functional understanding of how projects are conducted. This knowledge includes the steps of a typical outcomes assessment project, what must be done in each step, and who is responsible for getting it done. Staff members should be familiar with, if not proficient at, all of the various technical skills required to carry out an outcomes project. These include

- project design;
- project management;
- instrumentation;
- data entry;
- data quality control;
- statistical analysis; and
- feedback to clinicians.

Perhaps the most important new information to convey to the staff is not a set of skills but an orientation to the work. As has been discussed throughout this book, outcomes assessment should be defined primarily in terms of its unique mission for organizational change and a quantitative orientation to clinical care. A commitment to the mission must be instilled in the staff. To cultivate enthusiasm throughout the organization, each person on the outcomes assessment staff needs to become a champion for the concepts and an innovator for the methods. Some "unlearning" may be needed as, for example, clinical researchers or quality assurance professionals become involved in outcomes assessment.

Since outcomes assessment is a developmental undertaking, all members of an outcomes assessment team should possess general research and development competencies. These include

- communicating (both written and oral);
- organizing;
- problem solving;
- questioning;
- listening;
- innovating; and
- maintaining a tolerance for ambiguity.

The outcomes staff should regard itself as an internal consulting group and coaching team to the clinicians. Technicians must learn to be responsive to the customer and explain themselves clearly. Project coordinators must learn how to get work done through cooperation rather than through exercising authority.

How. There is no core curriculum for outcomes assessment education. We have developed a variety of informal and semiformal means of conveying the mission, the concepts, and the functional framework to our staff members. Most sites conduct topical seminars, journal clubs, and structured discussions on an ongoing basis. Relevant conferences may provide valuable educational opportunities. Some of us have established resource libraries containing relevant books, journals, and articles. Documentation of specific projects can be used as case studies to illustrate general principals of outcomes implementation.

Staff education, however, is largely informal and on the job. By participating in specific projects, staff members learn from each other and from other individuals involved in the work. Each central staff member should experience all phases of a project first hand to understand how the various tasks and functions interrelate. It is important that time be made available for staffers to compare experiences across projects.

Examples. In the process of developing a climate for outcomes assessment at the **Cleveland Clinic**, it was important to educate key persons in the state of the art. The directors of quality management and of quality research attended various seminars and workshops targeted at outcomes assessment and clinical applications of continuous quality improvement. Participating in an outcomes consortium of the American Group Practice Association gave them an opportunity to learn together with their counterparts from other health care institutions, and to benefit from the expertise of InterStudy and the pioneering work of New England Medical Center and Park Nicollet.

At **St Vincent**, most outcomes staff education comes through regular staff meetings and brown bag lunch meetings. Held once or twice per month, the "brown bags" allow staff to present work in progress to each other. Senior administrators within the St Vincent system are asked to give periodic updates on the current health care environment and other activities within the system.

Training

The core outcomes staff need skills training primarily in the various technological components underlying the outcomes program, for example,

- how to administer a questionnaire or conduct a mailed survey;
- how to enter data into the outcomes database;
- how to use the statistical software package; and
- standard procedures for responding to inquiries about the outcomes program.

How. The central outcomes staff for most sites will not be large enough to warrant formal skills training programs. It is important to document all routine functions in a reference notebook, and to make this reference readily available to all.

Example. Every **St Vincent** outcomes staff member is expected to attend at least one external training session per year at hospital expense. Staff conduct targeted training sessions on software tools or statistical techniques as demand is expressed within the group.

Awareness Raising

The outcomes staff should be a key resource in raising awareness of outcomes assessment throughout the organization. To do so, they must obviously be kept informed of the status of all internal projects. In addition, they should keep abreast of outcomes activities at other organizations.

How. Most outcomes programs are small enough for everyone on the central staff to have a working knowledge of all ongoing projects. As with other sorts of programs, it is important to provide opportunities for internal discussion that are both formal (staff meetings) and informal (impromptu discussions).

Raising staff awareness of the broader outcomes scene requires more planning. Program managers should nurture informal network ties with their counterparts at other sites. Staff should be encouraged to attend relevant conferences. There are several newsletters on the market that regularly feature outcomes assessment activities.*

consensus

The opportunity for us to share our experiences in the Outcomes Implementation Network has been extremely valuable to us. Efforts should be made to extend and to expand the network. This is discussed further in Chapter 6, Interinstitutional Issues.

Example. **St Vincent** conducts an annual off-campus outcomes retreat to reestablish focus for the coming year.

CLINICIANS

Clinicians are defined generally as those individuals responsible for delivery of care, such as physicians, nurses, rehabilitation personnel, pharmacists, and health educators.

---

* *Outcomes Measurement & Management* is published bimonthly by The Zitter Group, San Francisco. *Report on Medical Guidelines & Outcomes Research* is published biweekly by Capitol Publications Inc., Alexandria, VA.

Education

Clinicians should "own" the outcomes assessment initiative. A key responsibility of the outcomes staff is to help clinicians incorporate an outcomes perspective in their practice. This means educating staff in what may be broadly construed as quantitative thinking:

- Recording clinical information systematically.
- Asking good questions of the data.
- Interpreting statistical analyses.
- Using analyses to improve clinical treatment and decision-making processes.

How. As a rule of thumb, formal classes in outcomes assessment for clinicians do not work. Doctors are often unable or unwilling to make time in their schedules to attend sessions on what they perceive as having only tangential relevance to their practice.

We have had much better experience using specific outcomes projects as learning environments for clinicians. The various phases of a project provide a living laboratory to develop quantitative thinking in a personally relevant context.

consensus

In initiating an outcomes project, make sure that the participating clinicians commit themselves to being active collaborators. They should be given ample opportunities for involvement in project design and management. Data feedback should be explained and discussed interactively with the physicians.

Examples. At **Henry Ford Health System**, diffusion of outcomes assessment ideas and information is accomplished in part through a monthly newsletter distributed to all clinicians and key management leaders.

In 1991 Dr Sheldon Greenfield, a leading outcomes researcher, conducted a full-day program for key clinicians at **Cleveland Clinic.** Attendees included a few physician champions for outcomes assessment, as well as several curious physicians, nurses, researchers, and administrators. The RAND Corporation's (Santa Monica, CA) Medical Outcomes Study and implications for use of outcomes data in clinical practice were the core themes. This program was followed by several grand rounds presentations of early data from Cleveland Clinic's total hip replacement outcomes project.

With grant funding, **St Vincent** has developed a just-in-time approach to physician education. Groups of clinicians meet to discuss a specific clinical or practice problem and be introduced to outcomes and health status assessment as a tool for addressing the problem. In addition, the St Vincent Center for Outcomes Research and Education (CORE) has set up a Quality and Outcomes Reading Area for clinicians in the hospital library. This resource includes display journals, notebooks of relevant materials, reprint files, and a computer database of downloaded MEDLINE abstracts of relevant literature.

Training

Clinicians participating in a specific outcomes project must be taught their responsibilities in the project protocol. Key components of the clinician's protocol might include

- patient inclusion criteria;
- when and how to complete clinician data forms; and
- what to do with the completed forms.

How. The project protocol should be formalized, documented, and distributed to all participating clinicians. There should be a brief initial training session. Periodic feedback sessions should include discussions of clinicians' experiences in adhering to the protocol and how to make the process better.

consensus

If the clinicians own the project, they should also own the protocols. They are responsible for the quality of the data. Be prepared to revise the protocol if the physicians cannot make it work.

Awareness Raising

Clinicians as a group need to internalize the mission and vision of outcomes assessment if a program is to succeed. Some may already share the vision; others are amenable; a minority may be hostile. At a minimum there must be an ongoing, organizationwide awareness-raising campaign that conveys the purpose of outcomes assessment as it relates to clinical care. Other information must be tailored to clinicians with different levels of commitment.

- **The enthusiasts.** There will be clinicians who like the idea of outcomes assessment, are innovative, have some experience with data collection, and wish to become involved in an outcomes assessment project. These individuals will benefit from an awareness-raising experience that is more content-rich and educational in nature. Topics appropriate for the enthusiasts include
  - appropriate expectations of outcomes assessment;
  - history and goals of specific outcomes projects;
  - the project implementation process;
  - a general overview of methods;
  - interpretation of findings; and
  - closing the loop between outcome and process.

  The enthusiasts also benefit from peer support and the opportunity to explore ideas with their colleagues.
- **The empiricists.** Some clinicians are very research oriented and are willing to look at outcomes assessment if it generates data relevant to issues they are already pursuing. This

group can benefit from conceptual discussions in which the outcomes assessment staff introduces its instruments and methods for consideration.

■ **The rest.** This includes skeptics and those too busy to participate in outcomes assessment projects. This group needs more information about why outcomes assessment is becoming an increasingly important concern in health care generally, and how it is likely to affect them individually.

How. There should be a structured forum in which the strategic aspects of the outcomes assessment program—purpose, relation to broader organizational mission, activities to date, project roll-out time lines—are made known to all the clinicians. This broad public relations campaign should be directed to the least common denominator, not just to enthusiasts. It should include a rationale, targeted to skeptical and busy clinicians, as to why and how outcomes assessment will become increasingly important to clinical practice. Open discussion should be encouraged.

Examples. The **St Vincent** CORE director makes frequent presentations at medical staff meetings. Physician-to-physician communications regarding outcomes at hospital grand rounds have also been effective. Representatives of managed care companies have occasionally been invited to speak with clinicians about outcomes.

A major awareness-raising event at **Henry Ford** was a one-day conference on outcomes assessment held in September 1992. The conference, attended by more than 100 senior physicians and managers, presented the possibilities for outcomes studies, showcased achievements to date, and helped develop a long-term outcomes plan at Henry Ford.

PROJECT SUPPORT STAFF

Project support staff include the people responsible for performing the data collection and data entry functions for an outcomes assessment project. These may include waiting room receptionists, clinical technicians, nurses, and physicians, as well as central clerical staff dedicated to outcomes assessment.

Education

To the extent that these individuals' participation in outcomes is limited to their very specific roles in protocol adherence, their need for broader education in outcomes is minimal. However, most people want to know why they are being asked to do something and how they are contributing to the larger goal. An educational orientation helps capture their interest, builds their enthusiasm, and enables them to deal with patient and clinician resistance.

Example. At **St Vincent**, office staff are typically oriented to the outcomes field with a brief (one hour) presentation from CORE staff at the beginning of a project. The presentation includes discussion of the economic environment, concerns about medical quality, and illustrative data from successful outcomes assessment projects.

Training

To do their work effectively, project support staff must be trained in the specifics of the project's data protocol—the nuts and bolts for implementing a project. These include

- when and how to select eligible patients;
- when and how to administer patient self-report forms;
- when and how to collect clinical and laboratory data;
- when and how to follow up for missing data;
- who to ask when questions arise;

- where to send the completed data forms; and
- how to enter data into the database.

How. To accomplish concrete skills training, most sites use a structured walk-through of the protocol. At the beginning of a project, all persons responsible for protocol compliance are presented with formal documentation of the protocol: patient selection criteria, copies of the instruments, follow-up procedures, and data flow diagrams. Then the project coordinator walks the support staff through each step of the protocol, explaining the requirements and responding to questions. Throughout the duration of the project, the coordinator remains responsible for explaining modified protocols and training new staff on an as-needed basis. Project support staff should be given frequent opportunities to discuss problems with the protocol and to look for possible improvements.

ADMINISTRATION

Administration refers to the authority figures in a health care organization. Included are both nonclinical and clinical managers, as well as persons with both formal and informal influence within the organization. These people are key to the programmatic success of outcomes assessment.

Awareness Raising

For outcomes assessment to succeed, administrators must support the program in tangible ways. Resources must be made available; clinicians should be encouraged, and possibly compensated, to participate in projects. To make this sort of commitment, administrators need to understand the importance of outcomes assessment. In particular, there must be bridges built between the specific goals of outcomes assessment and the broader mission and strategy of the organization. Linkages should be emphasized between outcomes assessment and quality of care, cost containment, marketing and purchaser demand, patient centeredness, and relations with clinicians.

How. In our experience, administrators are best informed via fairly formal means of communication. Focused memos and presentations can be used to update top management on progress to date. The outcomes director needs to be proactive in explaining the work of the program and why the work is important to the organization. Administrators tend to pay attention to such rationales as purchaser expectations and physician relations. Marketing personnel may benefit from establishing a structured process for obtaining updated information on specific outcomes projects. The outcomes director should also seek to secure a seat in the formal venues for organizational strategic planning.

Informal awareness raising, though necessary, is probably most effective when not consciously orchestrated by the outcomes team. Word of mouth from enthused clinicians and purchasers has more influence than a targeted campaign.

Examples. At **St Vincent,** the CORE has established an executive committee. Consisting of senior administrators, the committee receives a briefing on one major outcomes project per month.

Cleveland Clinic draws attention to outcomes assessment in the context of practice guidelines. The view that credible outcome measures are needed to identify best practices and evaluate guidelines has growing support among clinicians and administrators.

PATIENTS

Education

Most of us are exploring ways to provide patients with feedback about their health status and outcomes of care. For this feedback to be useful, patients must be taught how to use the information in evaluating their health, the effectiveness of their care, and the decisions they need to make.

How. Patient feedback is a new phase in our work, so we have little experience on which to make recommendations. The interactive videodisk technology implemented by Jack Wennberg's group at Dartmouth Medical School (Hanover, New Hampshire) offers an intriguing possibility for giving patients information about expected outcomes of alternative treatments. Equipped with relevant data, patients can make more informed decisions about which treatments to choose.

Example. At **St Vincent**, many patients asked to complete follow-up surveys by mail. In addition to a questionnaire, the mail-out packet includes a newsletter about outcomes that is written for a lay audience.

Training

Patients have an important role in the success of an outcomes project: They must complete health questionnaires accurately. Patients should be made aware that their cooperation in providing key information about their health is part of their responsibility in maximizing the effectiveness of their care.

How. Whoever is responsible for questionnaire distribution should give brief verbal instructions to the patient. The clinician should reinforce to the patient the importance of the data.

KEY EXTERNAL PARTIES

Various constituencies outside the health care system need to be informed about outcomes assessment:

- Insurers;
- Purchasers; and
- Regulators: government, accreditation agencies.

Education

Insurers, purchasers, and regulators are often encouraged to make inappropriate uses of outcomes data. We believe that the health care organization should take a proactive role in teaching insurers and purchasers to be responsible consumers of outcomes information. Useful knowledge for consumers includes

- how to interpret data reports;
- understanding variation and its causes;
- interpreting comparisons of outcomes between sites;
- how clinicians use outcomes to improve the care process; and
- the importance of data confidentiality.

How. If these external customers want access to data, the outcomes group should establish a forum for open discussion of the key issues. Clinicians and administrators should be encouraged to participate.

Awareness Raising

Important external customers are key to organizational support of outcomes assessment. In the long term, outcomes assessment will be of direct benefit to anyone who must make decisions about the effectiveness of routinely delivered care. This long-term promise, as well as realistic short-term expectations, must be communicated.

How. The outcomes program's communication with the broader community is typically indirect. Marketing and development personnel must be taught the basics of outcomes assessment from a consumer's standpoint. When opportunities present themselves, the outcomes director should make formal presentations to consumer groups and payers. The outcomes team should also be responsive to customers' and regulators' requests for information about the program.

Example. The vice president for business and labor relations at

Henry Ford Health System is working with third-party payers and interested employers to help define the direction and intensity of Henry Ford's outcomes assessment activities. The employers are also being asked to consider the collection of outcomes data as "just another laboratory test" that should be reimbursable.

5
Ethical and Legal Concerns

Outcomes assessment is a new endeavor, with many of its promises and pitfalls yet to be revealed. Emerging from the work of the early demonstration sites are a number of ethical and legal issues affecting the outcomes team, clinicians, patients, and administrators. In most cases there are no clear answers, sometimes not even a clear consensus of opinion. This chapter identifies some of the issues that have arisen at our sites, along with our opinions about some of them. New outcomes programs should be aware of these ethical issues and give them thought before proceeding too far down the path.

consensus

The opinions we have put forward in this section should not be construed as conclusive legal opinion. Legalities are influenced to a great extent by state laws and specific circumstances. Seek legal counsel as is appropriate.

DATA ACCESS

Access to outcomes data is already a real concern, dating at least to the first release of hospital-specific mortality statistics by the Health Care Financing Administration. Who owns the outcomes data collected at a health care institution? Who controls the release of data and analyses to internal or external audiences? To whom, and in what form, should the data be made available? Again, there are more questions than definitive answers.

Data Ownership

Ownership is a legal construct. It is unclear who "owns" the data collected in an outcomes assessment project.

- Is it the patient, who is the central focus of care and of data collection? Certainly patients are the ultimate source of all data on their own health. Patients have the historic right to privacy and control over personal information.
- Is it the clinician, who usually controls access to the patient for purposes of data collection? Outcomes data must be interpreted from a clinical perspective if they are to be useful for decision making.
- Is it the outcomes assessment program, where primary responsibility for data management lies?
- Is it the institution in which the outcomes program resides? The institution typically owns the medical record, with clinicians and patients having specified mechanisms for gaining access to the record.

consensus

Seek legal opinion regarding data ownership.

Data Access/Management

In our experience, it is especially important to identify who has the power to control access to the data. Clinicians clearly control the front of the data stream. All the network sites have relied on voluntary cooperation of provider groups in initiating projects. All collect baseline patient data at the time of an encounter. All gather some patient-specific data directly from the providers. If the clinicians do not want a project to succeed, there are many places where they can shut off the data pipeline, or at least slow it to a trickle.

The health care institution housing the outcomes program has the potential to control the back end of the data stream. To date, however, the network members' institutions have not exercised this option. The health care delivery system is a loose and uneasy alliance of individual clinicians with the sites at which they deliver care. Administrators generally regard the physicians as their customers, who respond better to kid gloves than to a heavy hand.

consensus

> In practical terms, the outcomes program manager
> exerts the greatest degree of control over the data.
> The outcomes program is service oriented; in conjunc-
> tion with its customers, including patients, clinicians,
> and the institutional administration, the program
> should establish criteria to judge which requests for
> data should be honored.

Who Has Access?

Beyond *control* of access is the *right* of access. Not everyone has an equal need-to-know right to the outcomes data, analyses, and reports.

consensus

> Each institution should establish a legally defensible
> policy regarding release of outcomes-based informa-
> tion. The policy should specify the following:
> 1. Which types of *people* can have access to
>   information (for example, clinicians, administra-
>   tors, quality assurance departments, patients,
>   purchasers, regulators, the media);
> 2. Which types of *information* are covered by the

policy (for example, data, analyses of the data, reports of the analyses); and

3. What levels of *aggregation* of information are covered by the policy (for example, patient-specific, clinician-specific, and organizationwide outcomes information).

When questions arise, the outcomes program manager should defer to organizational policy on all data requests.

Confidentiality

The patient, the clinician, and the organization all have confidentiality concerns.

■ **The patient.** An organization should ensure that no outside party can identify a patient, even indirectly, from outcomes data. In this regard outcomes data are the same as any other information provided by a patient during the course of care.

■ **The clinician.** Physicians have a fear of being punished for what appear to be poor outcomes. We typically give clinicians feedback comparing their individual results with organizationwide aggregate results. Clinician-by-clinician comparisons are avoided unless there is consensual agreement among all participating clinicians.

■ **The organization.** Administrators fear that outcomes data might be used against their organization by competitors, purchasers, or the media. Again, release of information must be internally controlled.

consensus

The organization's data access policy should explicitly acknowledge rights of confidentiality and provide safeguards to ensure these rights.

Communication of Data Access Policy

Each network site's policies for data release have been pieced together in response to local conditions and specific circumstances. In each case, policy is based on the general consensus of the outcomes director, the clinicians, and the institutional administration. It is important to make all key constituents aware of the issues and to get their agreement on appropriate practices. Ideally this consensus building will be well underway before the first pilot project is begun.

Discoverability

To what extent is a health care organization legally *required* to release outcomes data? Are the data discoverable in the same sense that a patient's medical record may be subpoenaed during a lawsuit? This issue becomes moot if the outcomes data are in fact regarded as part of the medical record. Network members were divided on this issue.

- It is part of the mission of outcomes assessment that the data be used in routine medical care. The type of data collected is no different in kind from what has historically been included in the medical record. Logistically, it is desirable for the outcomes data forms to replace portions of the medical record. Therefore, it seems like a good idea that the outcomes data be made part of the record.

- Outcomes assessment is a developmental undertaking. For the most part, uses of the data in clinical practice are unknown. Clinicians are unfamiliar with the types of data recorded, and may lack confidence in their validity. Further, the statistical analyses of outcomes data are new to the clinicians; they may not know how to interpret these analyses in the care delivery context. Ultimately outcomes information should become part of the medical record, but this should happen gradually. For now, it may make sense to regard routine outcomes assessment as research, with the data kept separate from the medical record.

■ Another possibility is that outcomes data be regarded as part of quality assurance. There are some legal safeguards against discoverability of peer review documents.

Legal counsel at one of the network sites was asked to comment on the discoverability of outcomes assessment data. He noted that the Uniform Health Care Information Act, adopted in some states, regards all information given by a patient during treatment as equally discoverable. Information is protected as quality assurance documentation only in the context of facilitating free discourse among peers about possible quality problems. In practice, the *discussion* about quality is protected, but the quality *data* are discoverable.

consensus

Each organization faces unique circumstances.
Consult legal counsel regarding discoverability.

INFORMING THE PATIENT

What should patients be told about the potential uses of and audiences for the data they provide about themselves? To date we have stressed to patients that their participation is entirely voluntary. However, if the data come to be used in clinical decision making, patients' refusal to provide data may compromise their care. The issue of informing the patient needs continued attention as outcomes assessment programs mature.

Clinical Responsibility

Patients have reason to believe that all the information they give their physicians will be used in making treatment decisions. It is our hope that outcomes assessment data will be useful for and used in clinical decision making. However, there is a potential down side: A clinician who fails to act on relevant information could be held liable for a patient's poor outcome.

Since outcomes assessment is in the early developmental phase, the clinical value of the information remains unsubstantiated. As outcomes assessment becomes routine and establishes its value, it becomes part of the standard of care. That is, the monitoring and analysis of outcomes will become an essential part of patient care, and must be used with all patients in all conditions for which it is relevant.

consensus

Patients should be informed of whether, how, and when the outcomes information they provide will be used. Likewise, all clinicians participating in an outcomes project should understand the actual and potential uses of the data and analyses.

Responsibility of the Patient

Ultimately, physicians will use patient-reported outcomes data in clinical decision making (in some cases, physicians are already using this data). In that event, patients' responses to the questionnaires may have a material effect on their care. To ensure high-quality care, the patient must answer questions as accurately as possible.

Patients should be told that their responses are important. They should be encouraged to answer the outcome forms with as much diligence and as accurately as any other questions they may be asked during the course of treatment.

consensus

We do not believe that, before asking any question, the physician needs to know how each possible

response will affect a patient's care. This is an unrealistic standard, to which no other single item in the
medical record is held accountable. Clinical decisions
are based on a pattern of findings, not on any single
indicator. All sorts of information are considered in the
decision process, from casual observations to rigorous
laboratory test results. Outcomes data simply are part
of the overall pattern of findings that the clinician
must evaluate as a whole in decision making.

Impact on Patient Benefits

In our experience most patients respond positively to outcomes-
assessment data forms. However, a few patients are wary about
business-related issues. Some may fear that their poor health status
will affect their rates or continued coverage under their health
insurance plan. They may even be afraid of losing their jobs. On
the other hand, workers' compensation recipients may fear that if
they appear *too* healthy, their continued receipt of benefits may be
jeopardized. Anxiety may be heightened when data are obtained
by the relatively formal means of a structured questionnaire.

consensus

Again, outcomes assessment data are no different
from other information obtained about a patient
during the course of care. All such patient-specific
information is kept confidential and patients should
be reassured of this fact.

Internal Review Board

Internal review boards (IRBs) dictate the nature of patient informed consent in experimental interventions. If an outcomes
assessment project is defined as a study or as a developmental
method of evaluating or informing patient care, does it require

approval by the institution's IRB? Some sites have answered this question in the affirmative, especially those that define outcomes assessment as a research undertaking.

On the other hand, the outcomes data collection forms are merely a means of obtaining information that should be part of routine documentation of a patient's condition. Likewise, retrospective chart review forms used in quality assurance programs do not require IRB approval. Why should outcome forms be held to a different standard?

consensus

Outcomes assessment is expected to become a component of routine care delivery. The overall outcomes program should be presented to the IRB for informal review. However, we do not believe that project-specific IRB approval is appropriate.

DISTORTIONS IN THE DATA

Data Quality Control

The outcomes assessment team should build safeguards into the data management system for detecting and correcting systematic biases in the data. It is not necessary to attribute these biases to malfeasance; honest mistakes happen more often than dishonest ones. Safeguards might include

- reviewing schedules and admissions records to identify eligible patients for whom data have not been collected;
- confirming self-report data with other sources (for example, discharge, re-admission, death records);
- retaining records deleted from the outcomes database in a temporary buffer to make sure that the deletion was not made in error; and

- building bias detectors into the instruments to protect against "response set" (for example, the tendency of some people to answer yes to every question).

Methodological Bias

Outcomes measurement methods rely heavily on patient self-report. What about patients who cannot complete the forms? The easiest answer is simply not to include them in the database and analyses. However, if these data are in fact used in care decisions, absence of data may skew the analyses and, worse, may compromise some patients' quality of care.

There are certain shared characteristics of patients who do not complete outcome questionnaires. These include

- a language barrier that prevents the patient from reading the form in English;
- physical impairment (such as loss of vision or the use of the hands);
- mental impairment;
- situational anxiety (for example, a patient facing open heart surgery in a few hours); and
- acuity of condition, where the patient is too ill to complete the form.

In other words, there may be a systematic bias in the method against the underserved and the seriously impaired. This bias may result in inferior care for entire classes of patients. It may also distort aggregate statistical analyses and inferences regarding effectiveness and appropriateness of care.

consensus

We are making significant efforts to include the underserved in outcomes assessment projects. For example, nurses or family members can help patients complete the questionnaires. Each outcomes project should devise alternative pathways for capturing patient data. However, we have not succeeded in eliminating methodological biases entirely. Continued progress must be made as outcomes assessment moves from developmental status into mature implementation.

Gaming the System

All data collection systems are subject to systematic distortion. An incentive to "game the system" exists when participants in the data collection process have reason to believe that the data will be used against them. Physicians may fear being singled out as bad apples; patients may fear losing their benefits; administrators may fear losing contracts.

Prevention is clearly the most powerful tool against gaming the system. Ideally all affected constituencies should participate in deciding how and by whom the data will be used. At the very least they should be informed about uses of the data.

6
Interinstitutional Issues

A clinic or hospital may wish to collaborate with other organizations in outcomes assessment to

- gain access to methodology and technical expertise (for example, instruments, statistical analysis, software) not readily available in one's own organization;
- learn from each other's practical experience in implementation;
- pool outcomes data;
- compare results; and
- develop and validate new methodologies and instruments.

Collaboration helps virtually everyone, from sites with substantial experience in outcomes assessment to those with no experience at all. Few organizations possess all the technical resources needed to conduct a complete outcomes project. No project is perfectly implemented; all can benefit from each other's successes and failures. In our experience, those health care organizations that have decided that outcomes assessment "doesn't work for us" tend not to be actively collaborating with other sites.

Various mechanisms have been established or proposed to facilitate interinstitutional collaboration, including resource centers, data centers, consortia, and user groups. This chapter identifies some of these collaborative mechanisms and discusses their strengths and weaknesses.

METHODOLOGICAL RESOURCES

Instruments

Instruments for measuring patient outcomes can be obtained from a variety of sources. One key resource is the clinical and health services research literature. Most researchers make their instruments freely available, especially when their studies have been supported by public grants. Many papers publish the measurement tools used in the study; in other cases the instruments are available by request from the authors.

consensus

> Published instruments typically have the advantage of having been validated empirically. Such research-based instruments are particularly valuable for comparative purposes because normative data usually accompany the instrument. However, we have found that some modification to a published instrument is usually required to meet the particular needs of a given outcomes assessment project.

InterStudy has compiled several instruments for use in measuring outcomes. Collectively called *TyPEs,* these questionnaires include both general measures (demographics, risk assessment, health status) and condition-specific instruments developed by clinical researchers around the United States. The TyPEs are made available for a nominal fee and have been used in scores of outcome projects.

consensus

> InterStudy should be commended for compiling and distributing these instruments. For the most part, however, these tools have not been validated, and no

norms are available. They are excellent first drafts, which most sites modify to suit their purposes.

There are also sets of outcomes instruments that are commercially available. They typically focus only on mortality and clinical complications, and are embedded in a turnkey system for data collection, analysis, and reporting (for example, MedisGroups, APACHE III). These systems have usually undergone extensive development and rigorous testing, and provide extensive user support.

consensus

The cost of turnkey systems is offset by the convenience of implementation. Nevertheless, they are "black boxes," that is, significant portions of the instrument scoring algorithms and the normative data are not made available to the user. By themselves, such systems do not support the core mission of outcomes assessment: to monitor patient health status as well as adverse events, to establish an empirical basis for clinical practice, and to use outcomes as a basis for improving processes. If these systems can be augmented with additional data on health status and care processes, and if users are allowed to look inside the black box, these commercial systems can offer significant value in outcomes assessment.

Databases

Outcome database resources are of two basic types: database management systems and data management centers. A few vendors have begun developing databases for use by health care organizations. These systems are built around customized database software. Some systems use scannable forms for data entry; others use more traditional manual entry interfaces.

consensus

Given the lack of consensus and stability in outcomes instruments, it will be difficult in the near future for vendors to make available a general-purpose outcomes database management system that does not require extensive project-specific customization.

A few data centers have been put in place for entering and analyzing outcome data submitted by subscribing health care institutions. To date, however, these either support a turnkey outcomes system (addressed in the previous section) or a specific *data pooling* project (for a discussion of data pooling, see pages 123–125).

Technical Support

A need exists for technical support for outcomes projects on several fronts:

- Literature search;
- Instrument selection and modification;
- Database design and creation;
- Data management;
- Data analysis, presentation, and interpretation; and
- Educational materials.

Most sites that lack adequate in-house expertise either contract on an ad hoc basis with outside consultants or discuss specific issues with peers at other sites by means of informal networking.

consensus

There should be a national resource—either a center or a clearinghouse—to provide technical support to outcomes assessment projects. It is unclear, however, whether such a resource could be self-sustaining financially during this early stage in the outcomes movement. Additional outside funds will probably be needed.

SHARING PRACTICAL EXPERIENCE

Conferences

For the past few years InterStudy has conducted national conferences and regional training classes on outcomes assessment. These meetings combine formal presentations with opportunities to discuss common concerns in a structured context. Some health care organizations with active outcomes programs, including Henry Ford, Park Nicollet, and St Vincent among the network sites, hold outcomes conferences periodically. Clinical professional societies have recently begun to incorporate outcomes assessment into their agendas. Among federal agencies, the Agency for Health Care Policy Research and the Institute of Medicine regularly sponsor outcomes-based conferences.

Interest Groups

An interest group is a semiformal mechanism for bringing people together to share their experiences and concerns on a particular topic. Theoretically an outcomes user group could focus either on a particular clinical condition or on a shared technical issue (for example, analysis techniques). So far the only outcomes interest groups are clinical in focus.

Some professional societies have established outcomes advisory committees. Their purpose typically is to make policy recommendations to the larger organization rather than provide an ongoing forum for discussion. Thus, these advisory committees are not true user groups.

InterStudy periodically surveys licensed users of its TyPE instruments to identify which organizations are conducting projects on which conditions. InterStudy also serves as a sort of network broker for persons seeking others with experience in outcomes implementation. To date, however, there has been no concerted effort to establish more formal user groups.

The American Group Practice Association has established condition-specific user groups in the context of several data pooling initiatives. Various communication media are employed to share experiences: meetings, training sessions, conference calls. These groups are organized to maximize benefits to the participants.

- Materials for discussion are circulated to participants prior to the meeting or conference call.
- A leader is designated to manage the group.
- The leader asks key persons in the group to give site-specific updates on project progress.
- Extensive documentation is circulated promptly following the group session.

consensus

There is a clear need for outcomes interest groups. The AGPA user groups provide an excellent foundation for a broader-based initiative for one segment of the health care delivery system. Data pooling does, however, require a high level of commitment and complexity; pooling should not be a necessary condition for the establishment of a user group. As with a technical resource center, it will be difficult to create a self-sustaining user group structure without the infusion of additional funds.

Journals and Newsletters

A few newsletters focusing on outcomes have appeared on the scene in the last couple of years. These publications typically include interviews and synopses from outcomes programs. Articles are brief, with an emphasis on reporting rather than analyzing. Other newsletters with broader agendas (for example, quality management, group practice, managed care) have begun to include pieces on outcomes assessment.

consensus

> We are beginning to see the need for a new publication on outcomes assessment, one that focuses in greater detail on the technical and practical aspects of implementation. Such a publication would fill the niche, presently unoccupied, between the research journals and the newsletters.

DATA POOLING

Scope and Purpose

Data pooling refers to the aggregation of outcomes data from multiple organizations using the same instruments and protocols. In most instances the pooling project is organized around the collection of data on a particular condition or treatment. There are two main purposes for this sort of pooling:

1. To accumulate a large data set, permitting more detailed analyses and enhancing the study of relatively infrequent events; and

2. To compare results of care across institutions.

To date, there are three main outcomes pooling efforts that are underway:

1. The Managed Health Care Association, in conjunction with

InterStudy, is pooling outcomes data from various managed care companies nationwide.

2. The AGPA is coordinating several condition-specific pools composed of member clinics.

3. The Academic Medical Center Consortium has begun multisite outcomes data pooling.

Components of a Pooling Project

The significant advantages of data pooling come at a price: added logistical complexity in implementation. Certain essential issues must be addressed:

- A mechanism must be established for coordinating the project.

- Criteria for participation in the pool must be established, including rules about when and how an institution may enter or leave the pool.

- All participating institutions must agree on a common set of instruments.

- All participating institutions must agree on a common protocol for sampling and data capture.

- A method and location for pooling the data must be established.

- Data quality control issues must be determined, possibly including site audits to ascertain protocol adherence.

- Agreement must be reached on who will conduct data analyses and what analyses will be performed.

- Rules must be established regarding information release, including data confidentiality, dissemination of analyses, and publication rights.

consensus

Data pooling is more difficult to implement than in-house projects. However, the added burden is offset by the opportunity to explore collaboratively the methodological and logistical issues of outcomes implementation.

Since outcomes assessment is in its early phases, there is no preexisting agreement about the best way to implement an outcomes assessment project. As early as possible, try to establish a method for identifying issues and working out disagreements in a mutually agreeable manner.

Project Management

Much of the effort in pooling is directed toward achieving consensus among participants. This bottom-up approach contrasts sharply with the multisite clinical trial paradigm, in which the principal investigator specifies the protocol, and all participating sites agree to follow it. However, the same degree of rigor and consistency is required in an outcomes assessment protocol as in a clinical trial: Sites must use a single protocol and staff must be trained in the same skills and activities. In an interinstitutional outcomes assessment pooling effort it is not always clear who is in charge. A multitude of parties is likely to be involved.

- Outcomes assessment specialists from various sites may initiate the project.
- A number of clinicians may become actively involved.
- A project coordinator may be designated or hired.
- A data center may be contracted to process the data.
- An outside researcher may be engaged to serve as an unbiased expert on technical matters.

consensus

For internal and interinstitutional projects alike, it is important that clinicians take ownership of the project as early in the project as is feasible. Technical and managerial specialists should serve in an advisory role to the clinicians participating in the project.

Decisions should be based on consensus of participating clinicians. However, given the difficulty of arranging meetings across a broad geographic area, it is important that managers and technical experts be delegated the authority needed to make decisions in a timely manner.

Finally, it should be noted that many of the advantages of data pooling can be attained by multiple sites agreeing to follow a common protocol, then comparing results with one another.

7
Demonstrating Value

We believe that outcomes assessment is a valuable undertaking. What will persuade those who are more skeptical? How do we justify the time, expense, and inconvenience associated with the measurement and monitoring of outcomes? This chapter focuses on demonstrating the value of outcomes assessment. The following dimensions must be considered:

- Who benefits from outcomes assessment?
- In what ways is outcomes assessment valuable?
- What are the barriers to perceived value?
- How can relevant parties be persuaded that outcomes assessment is of value?

THE VALUE OF OUTCOMES ASSESSMENT

The importance of outcomes assessment is implicitly stated throughout this book. Nevertheless, it is useful to list some of the benefits that have been demonstrated or at least proposed.

To Patients

- **Communication with the doctor.** Structured questionnaires give patients the opportunity to describe their health and symptoms systematically, continually, and in detail.
- **Informed decision making.** By knowing which outcomes

to expect, patients are better able to choose among alternative treatments.

- **Self-care.** Outcomes assessment relies heavily on patients' ability to describe their own health status. This approach is inherent in patient-centered care: Patients assume responsibility for monitoring their care, making decisions about their care, and actively following the care plan.

To Policymakers

- **Population health.** Surveys of health status can help evaluate the overall health of the nation.
- **Productivity.** Measures of functional status and impairment point to the impact of health care on economic productivity in the society.

To Purchasers

- **Demonstrated value of health care.** By evaluating outcomes of care, purchasers can make decisions regarding benefit structure and provider networks based on the value of care, not merely on cost.
- **Appropriate utilization.** Outcome measures provide evidence regarding what treatments are effective for what types of patients.
- **Population wellness.** Health status surveys of covered lives can indicate the need for and effectiveness of prevention programs.

To Administrators

- **Continuously improving quality.** Integrated with a continuous quality improvement program, outcomes assessment can identify opportunities for improvement and can measure the impact of changes in the process of care on patient health status.

- **Program evaluation.** New and existing services can be evaluated with respect to their impact on patient health.
- **Marketing.** The ability to monitor outcomes is becoming a competitive advantage in markets dominated by savvy purchasers.
- **Improved efficiency.** By integrating a well-designed outcomes assessment program into the clinical care system, redundancies can be reduced in utilization review, quality assurance, and information systems.

To Clinicians

- **Clinical expertise.** Outcomes analyses give clinicians a quantitative perspective on how treatment affects patients' health. This new perspective enhances clinical experience and intuition.
- **Self-directed quality control.** Outcomes assessment can replace much of the traditional quality assurance and managed care apparatus used for external second-guessing of clinicians' decision making and performance.
- **Job satisfaction.** The opportunity to learn is inherently satisfying to most clinicians.
- **Publication.** The opportunity to share what one has learned is also satisfying, and in many institutions fulfills an expectation for professional performance.

BARRIERS TO PERCEIVED VALUE

If an outcomes initiative is to be successful, hypothetical benefits must become a reality. However, fulfilling the promise of outcomes assessment is not always a smooth road. There are three primary obstacles to demonstrating the value of outcomes assessment: cost, fear, and indifference.

Cost

Outcomes assessment does entail significant costs. In Chapter 3, Financing, we identified the major cost categories of establishing and administering an outcomes program. In addition to direct financial costs, there is also the burden of data collection imposed upon clinicians and administrative staff. Attempts to reduce this burden (for example, via retrospective chart review) may detract from the larger mission of establishing a quantitative orientation to clinical practice. Health care administrators are understandably loath to add yet another administrative line item to their budgets.

Fear

Part of the impetus for outcomes assessment is also a barrier to its acceptance by clinicians. Some purchasers perceive that outcomes analyses will enable them to distinguish more readily between "good" and "bad" providers. This so-called buy-right movement has made providers wary of outcomes assessment as a possible punitive measure imposed upon them by outsiders.

Indifference

Clinicians may view outcome measures as information that is "nice to know," but not essential to their work. This is particularly true of patient-based measures that, compared with hard laboratory findings, may be regarded as inaccurate, repetitive of information already contained in chart notes, and not interpretable in a treatment context. Clinicians may also discount aggregate results of outcomes assessment projects because the work is rarely published in well-known peer review journals.

PERSUASION

Clinicians and administrators must be persuaded that the value of
outcomes assessment significantly outweighs the cost. Persuasion
is largely a matter of

- documentation;
- communication; and
- synergy.

Documenting Value

Measuring the impact of process is what outcomes assessment
is all about. How can the impact of the outcomes assessment
process be measured? To date, little has been done on this front,
largely because most outcome projects are still in early stages of
implementation.

Many of the purported benefits of outcomes assessment can be
measured by means of questionnaires or structured interviews.
Some sites have begun to ask patients their opinions of health
status questionnaires; the response to date has been strongly
positive. Perceptions of clinicians are less well documented and
will probably remain so until more projects start generating useful
analyses. Meanwhile, clinicians participating in outcomes projects
should be asked frequently whether their goals and expectations
are being realized.

The value of an outcomes information system, like the value of
other information resources, is difficult to quantify. In some
projects the clinicians have begun to use outcome data forms as a
substitute for portions of the medical record. A few organizations
have been able to persuade purchasers to use outcomes assessment
in lieu of traditional quality assurance data; the Joint Commission
on Accreditation of Healthcare Organizations supports this trend
as well. Advocates of outcomes assessment tend to be in the
vanguard of the automated medical record movement, which will
presumably increase the efficiency of clinical practice. However,

other industries have generally been unable to document increases in professional workers' productivity as a result of improved information systems.

From a business standpoint, it is unclear whether marketing efforts that focus on an institution's superior outcomes have been effective in increasing revenues. There does appear to be a move by purchasers to include at least the ability to monitor outcomes as a key criterion in contracting decisions.

consensus

There is an inherent tension between business and clinical motivations for outcomes assessment. Advocates should be cautious in overemphasizing one currency of value at the expense of another.

At some point outcomes assessment will need to document itself clinically in tangible cost-benefit terms. Perhaps the most celebrated quantitative justification for continuous quality improvement in a clinical environment comes from LDS Hospital, Salt Lake City. Feedback of outcome and process data to physicians has led to demonstrable and measurable improvements in quality, decreases in unnecessary procedures, and reduced rates of readmission and complications. It is hoped that these demonstrated benefits outweigh the substantial investment in information systems that permitted the quality improvement work to be accomplished.

consensus

Outcomes assessment is too early in its development to be expected to justify itself in terms of improved quality and reduced costs. Nevertheless, these are the long-term target indicators of value to clinicians, administrators, purchasers, policymakers, and patients alike. Impact on cost and quality should be foremost in the minds of strategic planners as they develop and implement outcomes programs. Outcomes assessment programs would do well to emulate LDS's example by making the benefits of their activities explicit and quantifiable.

Communicating Value

Chapter 1 addresses the importance of internal communication as a momentum builder. It is important to identify key opinion leaders who are advocates of outcomes assessment and to update them regularly on work in progress. Ongoing successes of the outcomes initiative should be disseminated throughout the organization.

Other communication channels operating at a macro level may be equally influential in persuading administrators and clinicians regarding the value of outcomes assessment. Powerful groups such as the American Medical Association, professional societies, the Joint Commission, and purchaser coalitions certainly create a climate in which outcomes assessment is becoming more evident.

Clinical research has begun to focus more attention on patient outcomes and health status indicators. This trend is having a positive effect on practicing clinicians' attention to outcomes. However, the clinical research community has not actively tried to convince clinicians of the value of outcomes assessment.

- Funding agencies and journals continue to show a strong bias in favor of academically based randomized trial research. As a result, outcomes assessment in community settings is underfunded and underdisseminated.
- Academic researchers and community-based clinicians seldom collaborate in studies. Published findings are rarely translated proactively by the researchers into applications

for day-to-day health care. Consequently the gulf remains fairly wide between research and practice.

consensus

Clinicians respect academic journals. If you can get your outcomes assessment work published, it is well worth the effort in enhanced credibility. Editorial boards, however, still have difficulty acknowledging the unique contribution of findings drawn from observational data routinely collected in community settings.

Synergy

At this stage, the outcomes assessment movement has neither the influence nor the evidence to launch a strong crusade on behalf of its demonstrable value to clinical care. In both the short and long run, it is probably more effective for outcomes assessment programs to work cooperatively with other leading-edge movements for improving quality and efficiency. Joint efforts should produce more dramatic results and more effective communication of those results.

The broader quality movement is building momentum in the clinical community. The outcomes assessment program should work closely with CQI teams and projects for developing local practice guidelines. There should also be a concerted effort toward changing or eliminating less effective, more burdensome quality activities traditionally present in health care organizations.

There is a widespread movement toward integrated information systems and the automated medical record. Outcomes assessment can help this work by helping clinicians define their information requirements. Outcomes assessment programs will also benefit in the long run. Real-time data collection and feedback will become possible, and data for analyses will be available more easily and less expensively.

Finally, outcomes assessment can both support and benefit from the push toward vertical and horizontal integration of health care systems. Outcomes data can provide a common, depoliticized language for clinicians to discuss their shared interests.

CASE STUDY: CLEVELAND CLINIC FOUNDATION

In general, one of the most powerful ways we have demonstrated the value of outcomes assessment to patients, purchasers, policymakers, administrators, and clinicians has been through our own behavior as role models. From the onset we were conscious of the multiple barriers and resistance to outcomes implementation, not the least of which was the softer nature of health status measures. Another obstacle was the absence of a process in health care delivery for obtaining, recording, and storing patient-based measures. These were the areas where we made a concerted effort to give our outcomes projects a fair chance for success.

We designed the data collection methods to provide up-front information and support to patients and their families. Although the outcomes questionnaires we were using were identified as self-administered, we chose to obtain our first (baseline) data set in person. Patients were handed a questionnaire with a cover letter from their physician. Patients were then given a brief description by one of our data collectors of the importance of including patients' perspectives in the evaluation of the quality of their care. The developmental nature of these (or any) questionnaires was discussed and their cooperation and assistance in future data collection solicited. We also emphasized the personal nature of the information we were requesting. In an early pretest of the tool, we had several family members offer to complete the questionnaire for the patient and/or debate the answers the patient had entered. We were concerned about the validity of mailed questionnaires if this situation continued. We compared the outcomes measures to blood tests: Certainly no one would expect their physician to diagnose and treat them by examining blood sent in from a family member or friend.

We believe that our personal approach has reinforced the importance of the average of 85% to 100% return rates for follow-up questionnaires among all the outcomes projects. We believe this represents some value placed on this process by the patients. We are doing something right, or perhaps it is because patients already valued the information and they have always wanted to communicate it to their caregivers.

We have worked toward a delicate balance between intellectual ownership and freedom to doubt among the clinicians. Initially we realized it was more like a "short-term lease with an option to buy." Early on, the clinicians did not have to commit any of their own or departmental resources to the projects, and they were hesitant to generate practice implications from the data. The value aspect we focused on here was the opportunity to be a leader in the outcomes assessment movement and to set benchmarks. The intellectual and scientific curiosity of the clinicians was reinforced by our systematic methods and attention to detail. We believe they initially demonstrated the value they placed on the process by providing and reinforcing access to their patients. Now we are receiving requests to start an outcomes project for them— our customers are coming to us.

Perhaps our greatest challenge was to establish a process for systematically obtaining patient-based data without interrupting the busy and complex flow of care delivery or frustrating patients and clinicians. The timing and enrollment procedures for early pilots underwent several revisions before we settled on a smooth and efficient method to access patients at a time when they were not overwrought about a pending test or procedure. To accomplish this type of access we arranged for our scheduling system to make an appointment for "Health Status" one half-hour prior to the patient's visit with the physician. This appointment appears on the reminder note mailed to the patient 10 to 14 days prior to the office visit. It takes place in the same area as the office visit (in a vacant office or a corner of the waiting room) and is not billed to the patient. This has provided us with a structure for scheduling the efficient use of our data collectors and the reassurance that we do not compromise the process by interrupting the flow of care. We also believe this scheduling has communicated and/or reinforced the importance of outcomes information to the patients, since it appears on their schedule as part of their care.

We have also had to address fears that outcomes assessment was putting the organization at risk. For example: What if the patients say they do not function any better and the physicians say they do? Are we encouraging the patients to be adversarial and sue? Our support from the clinicians early on helped temper this concern—we are not yet sure what those differences could mean, but the patient is our partner in finding out.

Appendix
Outcomes Implementation Workbook

Implementing a successful outcomes assessment effort demands talent, resources, and hard work. It also requires planning. This workbook highlights many of the key issues that should be considered during the planning process.

This workbook is written for health care organizations that have an interest in starting an outcomes initiative, as well as for those that have already begun implementation. It can be used in various ways:

- As a reality test for the clinician or administrator wanting to lead the charge for an outcomes effort;
- As a self-assessment tool for the outcomes manager to evaluate progress and to plan the next steps; and
- As a basis for focused discussion among administrators, clinicians, and implementation specialists involved in outcomes planning.

Each section of the workbook is based on a corresponding chapter in this book. The reader should refer to the appropriate chapter in the text for the rationale behind the various questions, important background issues to consider in responding to the questions, and, where appropriate, consensus opinions of the Outcomes Implementation Network members.

This workbook is not a comprehensive how-to manual for planning an outcomes initiative. Don't expect to be able to answer every question: It could take years and, in our experience, the answers are continually changing as we move forward. We do recommend, however, that you push yourself to arrive at conclusions to these issues. We also encourage you to revisit the workbook periodically to explore where you have been, where you are now, and where you are going in outcomes assessment.

NOTE: Since you may want to use this workbook more than once, we suggest writing your answers on separate sheets of paper.

INTRODUCTION

For each question in this section, explore the opinions of the various key constituencies and customers of your organization: administrators, opinion leaders, clinicians, insurers, purchasers, and patients, as appropriate.

1. How important are the following motivators for launching an outcomes effort in your organization?
    (rank in order of importance from 1 to 6)

    ______ Automated medical record
    ______ Continuous quality improvement
    ______ Pressure from competitors
    ______ Purchaser demand
    ______ Scientific interest
    ______ Other ______________________

2. What types of health care outcomes should be routinely monitored? (circle all that apply)

    Complications

    Cost

    Functional status

    Mortality

    Physiological indicators

    Satisfaction

    Signs and symptoms

    Well-being

    Other ______________________

3. Is your organization more interested in (check one)

    ❏ demonstrating that it has good outcomes? or
    ❏ continually improving its outcomes?

4. Is your organization more interested in (check one)

    ❏ preventing bad outcomes? or
    ❏ maximizing good outcomes?

5. Who is the best judge of health care outcomes? (circle one)

    Patients

    Payers

    Physicians

    Public policymakers

6. What is your organization administrators' general attitude
    toward change? (circle one)

    Resist change

    React positively to proven innovations

    Actively initiate change

7. What is your organization clinicians' general attitude toward
    change? (circle one)

    Resist change

    React positively to proven innovations

    Actively initiate change

Chapter 1. ORGANIZATION

1. **OPPORTUNITIES INVENTORY**
a. Which of the following outcomes-related activities are underway at your organization? (check all that apply below)

b. Can they form the basis for an outcomes assessment initiative? (check all that apply below)

c. Who are the key contacts for these activities? (fill in contact's name below)

Research projects that incorporate patient outcomes
❏ Underway ❏ Basis for initiative Contact: ______________________

Development of an automated medical record
❏ Underway ❏ Basis for initiative Contact: ______________________

A continuous quality improvement effort that involves clinicians
❏ Underway ❏ Basis for initiative Contact: ______________________

Purchaser demand for outcomes data
❏ Underway ❏ Basis for initiative Contact: ______________________

Expressed enthusiasm for outcomes assessment by clinicians and/or administrators
❏ Underway ❏ Basis for initiative Contact: ______________________

Implementation of MedisGroups, APACHE, or other turnkey data system
❏ Underway ❏ Basis for initiative Contact: ______________________

Other ______________________________
❏ Underway ❏ Basis for initiative Contact: ______________________

2. Does your organization's mission include the following? (check all that apply)

   ❑ A commitment to accountability
   ❑ A commitment to demonstration of value
   ❑ A commitment to high-quality patient outcomes

3. **HUMAN RESOURCES INVENTORY**

a. Does your organization have one or more of the following types of people essential for launching an outcomes project? (check all that apply)

b. Who are they? (fill in the name[s] of each individual{s})

   ❑ Individuals who are willing and able to assume leadership as a catalyst for the outcomes initiative
   Name(s): ____
   ❑ Clinicians enthusiastic about outcomes assessment
   Name(s): ____
   ❑ Top managers with at least moderate support for outcomes assessment
   Name(s): ____
   ❑ Individuals with research protocol design skills
   Name(s): ____
   ❑ Individuals with project management abilities
   Name(s): ____
   ❑ Individuals with other core competencies
   Name(s): ____

c. Can they be brought together in an outcomes assessment initiative?

4. Describe the following items for your organization's outcomes program.

   Program mission?

   Program strategy?

   Program scope (numbers and types of projects, and the like)?

5. What would you want your outcomes program to accomplish in one year? in five years?

6. What needs to happen (planning, commitment of resources, coordinated effort) to attain your organization's long-term objectives for an outcomes assessment program?

7. How do you want to define the outcomes group's function within the larger organization? Some possibilities (check all that apply):

   ❏ As an operating division or separate business unit
   ❏ As a service bureau, providing staff-level support functions
   ❏ As an internal consulting group
   ❏ As a source of leadership and advocacy group
   ❏ Other ___________________

8. Will your organization's administration encourage a grass-roots effort without insisting on tight control or immediate cost justification?

9. Is there an existing department or program that can provide a "good home"—protection without excessive control—for the outcomes initiative? Possible candidates (check all that apply):

   ❐ Clinical or health services research
   ❐ Quality assurance
   ❐ Continuous quality improvement
   ❐ Information systems
   ❐ Other ___________________________

10. How can you develop organizational structures and strategies that will encourage clinicians' ownership of the outcomes effort?

11. Who are likely candidates for managing the outcomes assessment effort?

12. Do you have access (either in-house or through consultants) to technical specialists needed for staffing an outcomes effort? (fill in name[s] of each technical specialist)

   Project design   ___________________________
   Project coordination   ___________________________
   Instrumentation   ___________________________
   Protocol specification   ___________________________
   Data collection   ___________________________

Data entry   ________________________

Data quality control   ________________________

Database management   ________________________

Statistical analysis   ________________________

Feedback and report
    generation   ________________________

Interpretation of results   ________________________

Linkage of data to
    care process   ________________________

Education and training   ________________________

Other   ________________________

13. Does a centralized or decentralized outcomes team fit best within your organization? (check one)

    ❐ Centralized   ❐ Decentralized

Chapter 2. PROJECT MANAGEMENT

1. PROJECT PRIORITIZATION

Have you devised a strategy or method for prioritizing potential outcomes projects?

For the following list of selection criteria for potential projects:

a. Rate the *overall importance* of each criterion (1 = not important, 5 = extremely important). Use this rating to apply to all potential projects, *then*

b. Rate the extent to which each *potential project* fits the criterion (1 = not at all, 5 = completely).

Criterion	a. Importance of Criterion / b. Project Fits Criterion					
Strategic importance						
Incidence of condition	a.	1	2	3	4	5
	b.	1	2	3	4	5
Frequency of encounters	a.	1	2	3	4	5
	b.	1	2	3	4	5
Cost of care	a.	1	2	3	4	5
	b.	1	2	3	4	5
Likely impact of data on	a.	1	2	3	4	5
care process	b.	1	2	3	4	5
Other strategic	a.	1	2	3	4	5
issues __________	b.	1	2	3	4	5
Interest of						
Clinicians	a.	1	2	3	4	5
	b.	1	2	3	4	5

	a.	Importance of Criterion
<u>Criterion</u>	b.	<u>Project Fits Criterion</u>

Interest of (cont.)

Administration	a.	1	2	3	4	5
	b.	1	2	3	4	5
Purchasers	a.	1	2	3	4	5
	b.	1	2	3	4	5
Other key parties	a.	1	2	3	4	5
	b.	1	2	3	4	5

Design

Related ongoing activities	a.	1	2	3	4	5
to build on	b.	1	2	3	4	5
Clarity of purpose	a.	1	2	3	4	5
	b.	1	2	3	4	5
Logistical simplicity	a.	1	2	3	4	5
	b.	1	2	3	4	5
Limited size and scope	a.	1	2	3	4	5
	b.	1	2	3	4	5
Measurement tools available	a.	1	2	3	4	5
	b.	1	2	3	4	5
Funding and other available	a.	1	2	3	4	5
resources	b.	1	2	3	4	5
Active participation of	a.	1	2	3	4	5
clinicians	b.	1	2	3	4	5
Other design	a.	1	2	3	4	5
issues ____________	b.	1	2	3	4	5

2. Do you have a strategy for maximizing the involvement of clinical departments in the following key aspects of outcomes projects? (check all that apply)

    ❏ Planning
    ❏ Design
    ❏ Data collection
    ❏ Data entry
    ❏ Data quality control
    ❏ Interpretation of results
    ❏ Use of results to improve quality of care

3. Have you identified members of the project team?
    (fill in the name[s] of project team member[s])

    Clinician leader ______________________________

    Project coordinator ______________________________

    Instrumentation specialist ______________________________

    Data collection ______________________________

       Clinician data ______________________________

       Patient data ______________________________

    Data entry ______________________________

    Data quality control ______________________________

    Database management ______________________________

    Data analysis ______________________________

    Feedback and reporting ______________________________

    Interpretation of findings ______________________________

    Other __________ ______________________________

4. Have you established consensus among participating clinicians regarding the main purpose of the project?

5. Do the project design and timeline include opportunities for piloting and redesign?

6. For each type of data you plan to collect, will you (check all that apply)

    ❏ Use existing measurement instruments?
    ❏ Adapt existing instruments?
    ❏ Create your own instruments?

7. Are the protocols for data collection and data entry well defined and readily implemented within the existing clinical process?

8. Do you have a quality control mechanism established to ensure data completeness and adherence to protocols?

9. Do you have a data analysis plan that is based on the stated goals of the project and is appropriate for the primary users of the findings?

10. Have you developed report formats that are appropriate for each potential audience?

11. How will the results be used to improve clinical care?

12. How do the project's database requirements fit with the organization's other information systems activities?

13. Are there other databases within the organization that are relevant to your outcomes assessment project and can you get access to them? (check all that apply below)

	Existing Relevant Database	Access to Database
Claims data	☐	☐
Registries (for example, tumor)	☐	☐
Quality assurance data	☐	☐
Pharmacy data	☐	☐
Laboratory data	☐	☐
Patient satisfaction data	☐	☐
Other ______________	☐	☐

Chapter 3. FINANCING

1. Do you have a reliable basis for estimating costs for outcomes initiatives? (check all those that apply)

    ❏ Prior projects
    ❏ Experiences at other organizations
    ❏ Pilot testing
    ❏ Other _______________________

2. In budgeting for an outcomes effort, have you distinguished start-up and technology development costs from the operating costs for managing specific projects?

3. **PROJECT BUDGETING**

    Use the following worksheet to put together cost estimates for specific outcomes assessment projects. You may want to develop a more sophisticated spreadsheet to help you arrive at total costs for each category.

Cost Category	Estimated Cost ($)
Planning and design	_______________________
Instrument development	_______________________
Data collection	_______________________
Database programming	_______________________
Data entry	_______________________
Data quality control	_______________________
Data analysis	_______________________
Report generation	_______________________
Interpretation of results	_______________________
Project management	_______________________

4. Can any of the costs for outcomes assessment be subsumed under other funded initiatives (for example, information systems, continuous quality improvement)?

5. What are the most likely sources of funding for outcomes assessment projects and infrastructure? (check all that apply) Do you have a plan for obtaining the necessary funds? (check all that apply)

	Source of Funds	Plan for Obtaining
Grants	❑	❑
Institutional fundraising	❑	❑
Consulting	❑	❑
Purchasers and insurers	❑	❑
General operating revenue	❑	❑
Special allowances from administration	❑	❑
Clinicians and clinical departments	❑	❑
Other _______________	❑	❑

6. Do you have a rationale and a plan for transferring most of the financing of outcomes assessment to the general operating budget?

7. Will in-kind time spent by clinicians and clinical staff be budgeted? Will it be reimbursed from project funds?

Chapter 4. EDUCATION, TRAINING, AND AWARENESS RAISING

1. Have you developed a standard "introduction to outcomes" presentation?

2. Do you have a communications plan for each of the following key customers of the outcomes initiative? (check all that apply)

   ❏ Clinicians
   ❏ Administration
   ❏ Patients
   ❏ Insurers
   ❏ Purchasers
   ❏ Other _______________________

3. Have you assembled a set of key articles and other materials about outcomes assessment?

4. Have you established a mechanism for keeping up with the state of the art in outcomes assessment: strategy, methodology, results, and so forth?

5. Do you have a method for categorizing clinicians in terms of their awareness, knowledge, and enthusiasm for outcomes assessment?

6. Are you equipping the clinicians with the ability to interpret outcomes data and use the results in improving quality of care?

7. Do you have a method for training support personnel in the data collection protocols?

8. Have you established both formal and informal means of disseminating the current status of outcomes projects within your organization?

Chapter 5. ETHICAL AND LEGAL CONCERNS

1. Do you have access to legal counsel?

2. Have you evaluated the pros and cons of including outcomes data and/or analyses in the medical record?

3. Do you have formal guidelines governing data access?

  a. Who has access (clinicians, patients, administrators, insurers, and so forth)?

  b. To what information do they have access (raw data, scored data, analyses, and so forth)?

  c. At what levels of aggregation do they have access (patient specific, physician specific, site specific, and so forth)?

4. Do you have a standard introduction to patient data forms that describes the purpose of the data and ensures confidentiality?

5. Are the clinicians in agreement as to whether outcomes data are experimental or part of routine care?

6. Have you discussed the outcomes initiative with your organization's internal review board?

7. Have you devised methods for capturing data from atypical patients (for example, non-English speakers, patients with physical or mental impairments)?

Chapter 6. INTERINSTITUTIONAL ISSUES

1. Have you identified those aspects of methodology or implementation that will require access to external expertise?

2. Do you make a point of interacting with people in other organizations that are involved in outcomes assessment?

3. If you are interested in pursuing a joint outcomes project, have you specified the objectives you hope to achieve?

4. Do you have access to a group of organizations that is interested in or already pursuing joint projects?

5. Have you considered the pros and cons of data pooling for your organization?

Chapter 7. DEMONSTRATING VALUE

1. Can you present a concise description of the value of outcomes assessment to each of the following key constituents? (check all that apply)

   ❐ Patients
   ❐ Purchasers
   ❐ Administrators
   ❐ Clinicians

2. How can you assure clinicians that their participation in outcomes assessment will not be used against them?

3. Do you identify, acknowledge, and document on a continuing basis the accomplishments of your organization's outcomes effort?

4. Do you have a method for communicating the successes of your organization's outcomes initiative to key constituencies?

5. Do you regularly ascertain whether participants and customers of the outcomes initiative are satisfied with progress to date and committed to future work?

6. Do you have a long-term strategy for quantifying the benefits of outcomes assessment?

7. How can your organization incorporate health outcomes assessment into its continuous quality improvement program?

8. How can your organization use outcomes measurement and monitoring methods in moving toward a structured and automated medical record?

Index

W